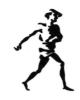

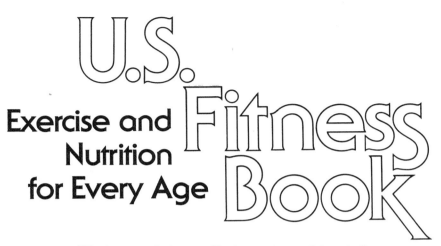

U.S.
Fitness
Book

Exercise and Nutrition for Every Age

Edited by PAT STEWART

Illustrated by JUDY FRANCIS

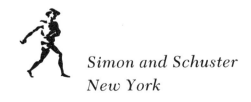

Simon and Schuster
New York

Published by Simon and Schuster
A Division of Gulf & Western Corporation
Simon & Schuster Building
Rockefeller Center
1230 Avenue of the Americas
New York, New York 10020

Designed by Irving Perkins
Manufactured in the United States of America

2   3   4   5   6   7   8   9   10

Library of Congress Cataloging in Publication Data

Stewart, Pat.
  U.S. fitness book.

  1. Exercise.   2. Physical fitness.   3. Nutrition.
I. Title.
GV481.S73   613.7   78-31609

ISBN 0-671-24678-X

Contents

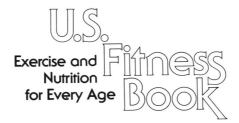

U.S. Fitness Book

Exercise and Nutrition for Every Age

Introduction

If you have decided that it is time to get in shape, you have a rewarding adventure ahead. The programs in this book are designed to help you condition yourself and achieve physical fitness on a sound, progressive basis.

Each program incorporates principles that can help you increase your strength, stamina, and flexibility; look, feel, and work better; and enjoy life to its fullest.

Like millions of adult Americans who recognize the virtues of physical fitness and would like to achieve it, you probably have wondered what to do, how to begin, how far to go. You may question whether you can spare the time, whether fitness is something that can be achieved by busy people with little time to spare.

These programs are designed so that you

will know exactly how and where to begin and what to do every step of the way. You will begin without strain or upset no matter how long it has been since you engaged in vigorous physical activity. In fact, they were designed for people who have *not* been exercising regularly! You will make steady progress toward a level of fitness that is best for you and that you will be able to maintain.

You will be able to measure your progress as you proceed. You will be able to exercise at home without special equipment and at a convenient time. And the time required will not be great.

Physical fitness can be achieved at any age. It does not happen overnight. It takes effort. But the feelings of well-being, renewed strength, and vitality are well worth the effort. Best of all, you can start on your way right now!

MORE AWARENESS THAN ACTION: A FEW WORDS ABOUT FITNESS

To look, feel, and be your best, you must exercise regularly. That is man's nature, and modern technology cannot change it. Few of us get enough exercise. Either our jobs or our daily activities do not allow it. When this happens, it is necessary to have a program of regular exercise. Your sense of well-being, your ability to perform, and even your survival depend on it.

You already know that regular, vigorous exercise increases muscle strength and endurance. It also improves the functioning of the lungs, heart, and blood vessels; makes the joints more flexible; relieves mental and physical tension; and helps to control weight.

Medical research shows that people who are active have fewer heart attacks than those who are not. When active people do have heart attacks, or get sick in other ways, they recover more quickly.

More than half of all lower back pain is due to poor muscle tone in both the back and the abdomen. In many cases, lower back problems could be prevented or even corrected by proper exercise.

In short, exercise can make the difference. The options are mere existence or a full life. The choice is yours!

WHAT IS FITNESS?

In a technical sense, physical fitness is a measure of the body's strength, stamina, and flexibility. In more personal terms, it is a reflection of your ability to work with vigor and pleasure, without undue fatigue, with energy left for enjoying hobbies and recreational activities and for meeting unforeseen emergencies. It is how you look and how you feel, and, because the body is not a compartment separate from the mind, it is also how you feel mentally as well as physically.

Physical fitness is many-sided. Basic to it are proper nutrition, adequate rest and relaxation, good health practices, and good medical and dental care. But these are not enough. An essential element is physical activity. Exercise for a body that needs it.

FITNESS IN AMERICA

Today's American adult is usually concerned about his or her physical fitness and is reasonably convinced that regular exercise is necessary for a healthy, vigorous life. Except for a dedicated minority, though, most people make only a feeble, irregular effort to exercise. They achieve little, if anything, in the way of fitness. Although several million Americans have taken up jogging (making it the most popular form of exercise in this country), about one-third jog only once or twice a week for about ten minutes.

Among Americans past fifty years of age, there is little awareness of the human need for physical activity. There appears to be a widespread belief that the need for exercise declines as one grows older. Some people believe that exercise beyond a certain age may be dangerous. A sizable majority of men and women past fifty do not exercise at all, and yet they seem to believe they are getting all the exercise they need.

These are highlights from the National Adult Physical Fitness Survey conducted late in 1972 by the Opinion Research Corporation of Princeton, New Jersey, for the President's Council. Here are some more specific findings:

• Forty-five percent of all adult Americans do not exercise.

• People who do not exercise are more inclined to say they get enough exercise than are those who do exercise. Sixty-three percent of the nonexercisers say they get enough exercise, while only fifty-three per-

cent of the exercisers believe they are as physically active as they should be.

• Of the sixty million American men and women who do exercise, nearly forty-four million walk, more than eighteen million ride bicycles, fourteen million swim, and fourteen million do calisthenics.

WHY EXERCISE?

Where there is muscle, there is need for exercise. The human body contains more than six hundred muscles. Overall, the body is more than half muscle. Muscles make every voluntary motion possible. They also push food along the digestive tract, suck air into the lungs, and tighten blood vessels to raise blood pressure when you need more to meet an emergency. The heart itself is a muscular pump.

Technological advances have changed our way of living. Strenuous physical exertion is largely unnecessary. The word "chore" has virtually gone out of use.

But the needs of the human body have not changed. Muscles are meant to be used. When they are not used, or not used enough, they deteriorate. If we are habitually inactive, if we succumb to the philosophy of easy living, we pay the price. Our bodies are less efficient. A growing conviction among physicians is that we are, to a great degree, what our muscles make us—weak or strong, active or inactive.

Offering strong support for this conviction

is the following observation by a former president of the American Medical Association: "It begins to appear that exercise is the master conditioner for the healthy and the major therapy for the ill."

A survey of nearly four thousand physicians showed that almost all of them now believe strongly that positive, healthy benefits, both physical and mental, accompany physical fitness resulting from regular, moderate exercise. It also showed that the great majority have come to favor the inclusion of tests of physical fitness in periodic health examinations and are convinced that physical-fitness programs, which have been largely aimed at children, are even more necessary for adults.

SOME BENEFITS OF EXERCISE

An obvious benefit of exercise is that flabby muscles are firmed. In addition, research shows that exercise helps vital organs to function properly—particularly the heart, lungs, and circulatory system. The heartbeat becomes stronger and steadier, breathing becomes deeper, and circulation improves. Research also shows the following benefits reported by people who, after a long period of sedentary living, start a systematic exercise program:

- Increased strength, endurance, and co-ordination
- Increased joint flexibility
- Reduction of minor aches, pains, stiffness, and soreness

- Correction of faulty posture
- Improvement in general appearance
- Increased efficiency with reduced energy expenditure while doing both physical and mental work
- Better ability to relax and reduce tension
- Less chronic fatigue

EXERCISE AND CHRONIC FATIGUE

One of the most frequently voiced complaints today is that of chronic tiredness. While it can stem from illness, research shows that most chronic tiredness is the result of too little exercise. Continual inactivity produces muscular atrophy, and the individual soon becomes under-muscled for his or her weight. There is not enough physical strength to work and play easily and efficiently.

One important end result of the increase in muscular strength and general endurance provided by exercise is an increase in the body's capacity for doing normal daily activities. The fatigue limit is pushed back. Valid research shows that a fit person uses less energy for any given movement or effort than a flabby or weak person.

EXERCISE AND THE HEART

The old-fashioned idea that exercise is bad for the heart is without scientific foundation. Actually, it has been proven that *appropriate exercise strengthens the heart*.

There is a growing body of evidence that

supports this fact. It includes findings of lower cholesterol levels in active people, faster clearing of fats from the blood after meals, and sharply reduced heart-attack rates.

A recent study of 120,000 American railroad employees showed that the heart-attack rate among the office workers was almost twice that of the men working in the yards. Other studies, in the United States, England, and elsewhere, also show a higher rate of heart attacks among those who do not have jobs that require them to be physically active. In addition, the studies indicate that when a heart attack does occur the physically active person is more likely to recover. One possible reason for this is that exercise may promote the development of supplementary blood vessels, which can take over the burden of nourishing the heart muscle when a coronary artery is blocked in a heart attack.

EXERCISE AND AGING

There is also strong support for the belief that regular exercise can help resistance to degenerative disease and slow down the physical deterioration that comes with age.

People who exercise regularly and consistently seem to have better job performance records, fewer degenerative diseases, and a longer life expectancy than people who do not exercise. Proper exercise can make the later years active years.

HOW MUCH EXERCISE AND HOW OFTEN?

The amount of exercise needed varies from one individual to another, but the American Medical Association recommends thirty to sixty minutes daily as a minimum. No one can achieve a satisfactory level of strength, endurance, and flexibility by working out only once a week. Daily exercise sessions bring about the best results.

The way in which an exercise is done is just as important as how often it is done. For best results, the individual must work hard enough to breathe heavily and "break into a sweat." People who are unfamiliar with human physiology or with the principles of exercise seldom work hard enough or long enough to improve circulatory and respiratory performance or to strengthen muscles. One reason for this is that many of our more popular and enjoyable participatory sports are not taxing enough for fitness purposes. They make a contribution but should be supplemented by an exercise program.

Dynamic good health is the objective of a physical fitness program. Performing exercises halfheartedly or working out briefly and sporadically cannot move you any closer to that goal. Hard work on a regular, sustained basis is the answer.

The level of fitness you can reach depends on your age, your body's built-in potential, and previous conditioning. It also depends on your state of mind. It is much easier to do something when you want to and believe you can.

When you begin your personal exercise

program, you should not expect dramatic overnight changes. But, gradually over the next weeks and months, you will begin to notice a new spring in your step, a new ease in carrying out ordinary daily activities. You will find yourself with more energy left at the end of the working day and new zest for recreation in the evening. Most likely, you will be sleeping more soundly than you have for years and waking more refreshed in the morning. In short, you will be on your way to a better and more complete life.

BEFORE YOU BEGIN

Before you begin any exercise program, it is a good idea to have a medical checkup. If you have not had an examination in the past year, if you are past thirty, if you are overweight, or if you have a history of high blood pressure or heart trouble, a medical checkup may help you to avoid very serious consequences.

Chances are your physician will give you an unconditional go-ahead. If not, he can modify the exercises so that they are suited to you. There are some people who should not undertake any exercise program. Only a qualified physician can say for sure if the exercise programs outlined here are advisable for you. Show him this book and ask his advice.

A FINAL NOTE

This book is designed for the whole family. As you read through the various sections, you will notice that some information has been repeated. This is done so that each section is complete. There is no need to flip back and forth among the different programs.

Getting Ready

HOW TO BEGIN

If your physician has not selected an exercise program for you already, the tests described here will help you make the right choices. They will measure your present exercise tolerance so you can decide at which level to begin the walking-jogging part of the program. This chapter will prepare you for the more strenuous programs later on. Remember though, no two people, even when they are of the same age, sex, and physical condition, have the same exercise tolerance. That is why your program should be based on *your* personal test results rather than on what someone else is doing or on what you think you should be doing.

A WORD OF CAUTION

If you develop nausea, trembling, extreme breathlessness, pounding headache, or chest pains while taking these tests, stop immediately. These symptoms indicate that you have gone beyond your present level of exercise tolerance.

If the symptoms do not pass within five minutes, discontinue the program and check with your physician.

WALK TEST

This test determines how many minutes (up to ten) you can walk at a brisk pace, on a level surface, without undue difficulty or discomfort. If you can walk for—

- five minutes or less, begin with the Level One walking program.
- more than five minutes, but less than ten, begin with the Level One walking program, Week 3.
- the full ten minutes, but are tired and sore, start with the Level Two walking-jogging program.
- the full ten minutes without discomfort, you are in shape for bigger things. Wait twenty-four hours and take the Walk-Jog Test.

WALK-JOG TEST

Walk fifty steps (left foot strikes the ground twenty-five times) and jog fifty steps for a total of ten minutes. Read the Jogging Guidelines (see page 33) before taking the test.

Walk at the rate of 120 steps per minute (left foot strikes the ground at one-second intervals). Jog at the rate of 144 steps per minute (left foot strikes the ground eighteen times every fifteen seconds). If you find that—

- you cannot complete the ten-minute test, begin with the Level Two program, Week 3.
- you can complete the ten-minute test but are tired and winded, start with the Level Two program, Week 4.
- you can finish the ten-minute test without difficulty, start with the Level Three program.

YOUR EXERCISE PROGRAM

The routines outlined here use the most up-to-date information available on exercise physiology. They are beneficial for both men and women. Follow the instructions carefully.

The program consists of three parts:

1. Warm-up
2. Conditioning exercises
3. Circulatory activities

The circulatory activities are divided (according to intensity) into three levels— Level One, Level Two, and Level Three. Level One is the least strenuous, and Level Three is the most strenuous.

The conditioning exercises will improve your muscle tone; increase your strength slightly; and improve your posture, flexibility, coordination, and balance.

The circulatory exercises will improve the efficiency and the capacity of your lungs, heart, and blood vessels.

General Advice

Start both the conditioning and circulatory routines by doing each exercise the minimum number of times shown. Gradually increase the number until you can do the exercise the maximum number of times with ease, and then go to the next level. As you move along, your exercise tolerance will increase.

For the best results, exercise daily. As you

begin to get into shape, substitute an equal amount of swimming, hiking, tennis, or dancing for the circulatory exercises several times a week.

In the early stages of the program, you may become stiff or sore; your feet and knees may hurt. If this happens, reduce or stop the walking-jogging part of the program until the soreness or pain disappears. Continue the warm-up or conditioning exercises. If the pain or soreness persists for several weeks, check with your physician.

Set up a regular routine. You should choose a convenient time and stick with it. No particular time of day is better than any other. You should take advantage of daily opportunities for additional exercise. When time permits, walk rather than drive. Take the stairs instead of the elevator. Practice bending, stretching, stooping, pushing, and pulling as you go through each day.

There is no easy way to keep fit. Reaching and keeping a satisfactory fitness level require long, vigorous exercise so that body temperature and heart and breathing rates increase. You have to sweat a little.

It is a good idea to set aside at least thirty minutes a day for planned exercise. If you do not, you may pay for it in time lost through illness or premature aging.

The Warm-Up

Before you start the conditioning or circulatory exercises, warm up your body. The following warm-up exercises will increase your breathing rate and raise your body temperature while at the same time your muscles will be stretched. These exercises concentrate on the lower back to help prevent problems in that area.

REACH AND BEND

Starting Position: Stand erect, feet shoulder width apart, arms extended over head.

Action: Stretch as high as possible, keeping heels on ground. Hold for a count of 15 to 30.

FLEXED-LEG BACK STRETCH

Starting Position: Stand erect, feet shoulder width apart, arms at side.

Action: Slowly bend over, touching the ground between the feet. Keep the knees flexed. Hold for a count of 15 to 30. If you cannot reach the ground at first, touch the top of your shoe line.
Repeat 2 to 3 times.

ALTERNATE KNEE PULL

Starting Position: Lie on back, feet extended, hands at side.

Action: Pull one leg to chest, grasp with both arms

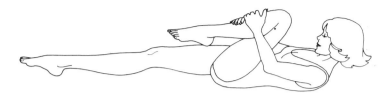

and hold for a count of 5. Repeat with opposite leg.

Repeat 7 to 10 times with each leg.

DOUBLE KNEE PULL

Starting Position: Lie on back, feet extended, hands at side.

Action: Pull both legs to chest, lock arms around legs, pull buttocks slightly off ground. Hold for a count of 20 to 40.

Repeat 7 to 10 times.

TORSO TWIST

Starting Position: Lie on back, knees bent, feet on the ground, fingers laced behind neck. For best result, place your feet under something to prevent them from lifting during action.

Action: Count 1. Lift torso to upright position and twist, touching the right knee with the opposite elbow.

Count 2. Return to starting position.

Count 3. Repeat, twisting in opposite direction. Exhale on the way up, inhale on the way down.

Repeat 5 to 15 times.

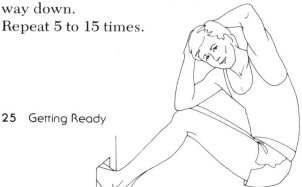

Conditioning Exercises

The following exercises constitute a basic all-round program.

Abdominal

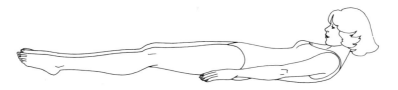

HEAD AND SHOULDER CURL (BEGINNER)

Starting Position: Lie on back, legs straight, arms at sides.
Action: Count 1. Lift head and shoulders off floor. Hold this position for 5 counts.
Count 2. Return to starting position.
Repeat 10 to 15 times.

SIT-UP, ARMS CROSSED (INTERMEDIATE)

Starting Position: Lie on back, arms crossed on chest, hands grasping opposite shoulders.
Action: Count 1. Lift up to sitting position.
Count 2. Return to starting position.
Repeat 10 to 15 times.

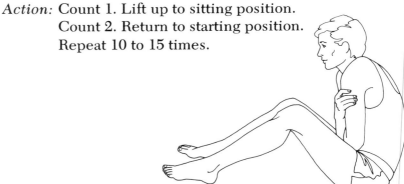

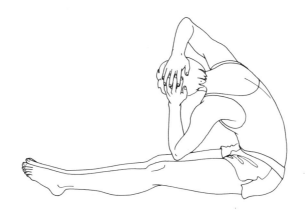

SIT-UP, FINGERS LACED (ADVANCED)

Starting Position: Lie on back, legs extended and feet spread one foot apart, fingers laced behind neck.

Action: Count 1. Lift up to sitting position and touch right elbow to left knee.

Count 2. Return to sitting position.

Count 3. Touch left elbow to right knee.

Count 4. Return to starting position.

Repeat 15 to 25 times.

Shoulder–Arm

HORIZONTAL ARM CIRCLES

Starting Position: Stand erect, arms extended sideways at shoulder height, palms up.

Action: Rotate hands and arms, clockwise. Turn palms down and rotate hands and arms counterclockwise.

Repeat 15 to 20 times in each direction.

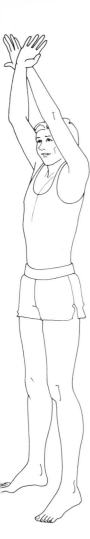

GIANT ARM CIRCLES

Starting Position: Stand erect, feet shoulder width apart, arms at sides.

Action: Raise arms straight up. Bring them together so that wrists cross. Lower arms to side. Repeat 10 times.

Arms and Chest

When doing these exercises, it is important to keep your back straight. Start with the knee pushup and continue for several weeks until your stomach muscles are toned up enough to keep your back straight. Then try the intermediate.

KNEE PUSH-UP (BEGINNER)

Starting Position: Lie prone, hands outside shoulders, fingers pointing forward, knees bent.

Action: Count 1. Straighten arms, keeping back straight.
Count 2. Return to starting position.
Repeat 5 to 10 times.

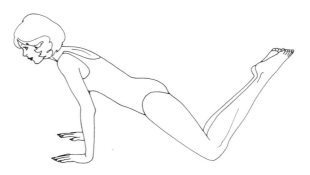

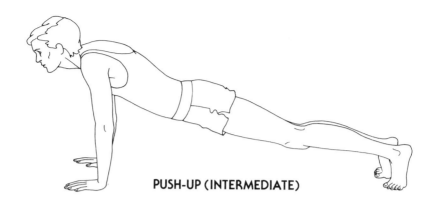

PUSH-UP (INTERMEDIATE)

Starting Position: Lie prone, hands outside shoulders, fingers pointing forward, feet on floor.

Action: Count 1. Straighten arms, keeping back straight.
Count 2. Return to starting position.
Repeat 10 to 20 times.

Lower Body

This sequence of exercises is designed to tone up your thighs, buttocks, and calves. Do each of them with every workout.

QUARTER KNEE BENDS

Starting Position: Stand erect, hands on hips, feet comfortably spaced.

Action: Count 1. Bend knees to 45°, keeping heels on floor.
Count 2. Return to starting position.
Repeat 15 to 20 times.

SITTING SINGLE LEG RAISES

Starting Position: Sit erect, hands on side of chair seat for balance. Legs extended at angle to floor.
Action: Count 1. Raise left leg waist-high.
Count 2. Return to starting position.
Repeat equal number with opposite leg.
Repeat 10 to 15 times for each leg.

SIDE LYING LEG LIFT

Starting Position: Lie on right side, legs extended.
Action: Count 1. Raise left leg as high as possible.
Count 2. Lower to starting position.
Repeat on opposite side.
Repeat 10 to 15 times for each side.

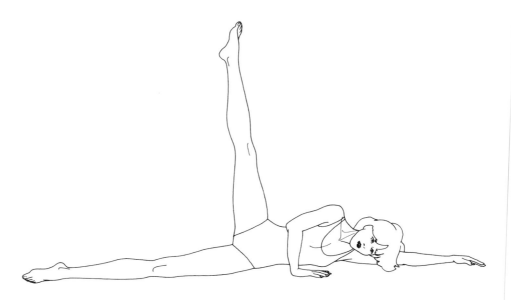

BACK LEG SWING

Starting Position: Stand erect behind chair, feet together, hands on chair for support.

Action: Count 1. Lift one leg back and up as far as possible.

Count 2. Return to starting position.

Repeat equal number of times with other leg.

Repeat 20 times for each leg.

HEEL RAISES

Starting Position: Stand erect, hands on hips, feet together.

Action: Count 1. Raise body on toes.

Count 2. Return to starting position.

Repeat 20 times.

Circulatory Activities

Level One Walking Program

Week	Daily Activity
1	Walk at a brisk pace for five minutes, or for a shorter time if you become tired. Walk slowly or rest for three minutes. Walk briskly for five minutes, or until you become uncomfortably tired.
2	Same as Week 1, but increase your pace as soon as you can walk for five minutes without becoming sore or tired.
3	Walk at a brisk pace for eight minutes or less if you become too tired. Walk slowly or rest

for three minutes. Walk briskly for eight minutes, or until you become tired.

4   Same as Week 3, but increase your pace as soon as you can walk eight minutes without becoming sore or tired.

When you have completed Week 4 of the Level One program, go on to Week 1 of the Level Two program.

Level Two Walking-Jogging Program

Week   *Daily Activity*

1   Walk at a brisk pace for ten minutes, or less if you become too tired. Walk slowly or rest for three minutes. Walk briskly for ten minutes, or until you become too tired.

2   Walk at a brisk pace for fifteen minutes, or less if you become too tired. Walk slowly for three minutes.

3   Jog twenty seconds (50 yards). Walk one minute (100 yards). Repeat twelve times.

4   Jog thirty seconds (75 yards). Walk 1½ minutes (150 yards). Repeat twelve times.

When you have completed Week 4 of the Level Two program, begin at Week 1 of the Level Three program.

Level Three Program

Week   *Daily Activity*

1   Jog forty seconds (100 yards). Walk one minute (100 yards). Repeat nine times.

2   Jog one minute (150 yards). Walk one minute (100 yards). Repeat eight times.

3   Jog two minutes (300 yards). Walk one minute (100 yards). Repeat six times.

4 Jog four minutes (600 yards). Walk one minute (100 yards). Repeat four times.

5 Jog six minutes (900 yards). Walk one minute (100 yards). Repeat three times.

6 Jog eight minutes (1200 yards). Walk two minutes (200 yards). Repeat two times.

7 Jog ten minutes (1500 yards). Walk two minutes (200 yards). Repeat two times.

8 Jog twelve minutes (1700 yards). Walk two minutes (200 yards). Repeat two times.

JOGGING GUIDELINES

How to Jog

Run in an upright position. Avoid the tendency to lean. Keep your back as straight as you comfortably can. Keep your head up so as not to look at your feet.

Hold your arms slightly away from your body. Bend your elbows so that your forearms are almost parallel to the ground. Occasionally shake and relax your arms and shoulders to help reduce the tightness that sometimes develops while jogging. Periodically take several deep breaths and blow them out to help you relax.

It is best to land on the heel of the foot and rock forward so that you drive off the ball of the foot for your next step. If this proves difficult, try a more flat-footed style. Jogging on the balls of your feet, as in sprinting, will produce severe leg soreness. Keep your steps short and let your foot strike the ground beneath your knee. The length of your stride should vary with your rate of speed.

Breathe deeply with your mouth open. Do not hold your breath.

If you become unusually tired or uncomfortable, slow down, walk, or stop.

What to Wear

Select loose, comfortable clothes. You should dress for warmth in the winter and for coolness in the summer. "Jogging suits" or "warm-ups" are not necessary, but they are practical and comfortable.

Do not wear rubberized or plastic clothing. Increased sweating will not produce permanent weight loss. Such clothing can cause your body temperature to rise to dangerous levels. Rubberized or plastic clothing interferes with the evaporation of sweat, the body's chief temperature-control mechanism during exercise. If sweat cannot evaporate, heat stroke or heat exhaustion may result.

Shoes with firm soles, good arch supports, and pliable tops are essential. Shoes made especially for distance running or walking are the best. Ripple or crepe soles are excellent for running on hard surfaces. Beginners should avoid inexpensive, thin-soled sneakers. It is important to wear clean, soft, heavy, well-fitting socks. Beginners may want to wear thin socks under the heavier pair.

Where to Jog

If possible, avoid hard surfaces such as concrete and asphalt for the first few weeks.

Running tracks (located at most high schools), grass playing fields, parks, and golf courses are recommended. In bad weather, jog in the protected area around shopping centers, or in your garage or basement. In the city try a school playground. Different locations and routes will add interest to your program.

When to Jog

The time of day for jogging is not important. However, do not jog within an hour of eating or during an excessively hot, humid day.

It is important, though, to commit yourself to a regular schedule. Some people believe that those who jog early in the morning tend to be more faithful than those who run in the evenings. People who jog with family members or friends also tend to stay with their jogging program. Companionship, however, not competition, should be your goal when jogging with someone else.

Illness or Injuries

Try to prevent blisters, sore muscles, and aching joints. If you are ill, ask your physician if you should jog. Any persistent pain or soreness should be discussed with your physician.

Women's Exercises

This program is designed for the woman who has not done any consistent, vigorous, all-around exercise recently. Housework does not fit this definition because only certain muscles are used on a regular basis. The program starts with an orientation, or "get-set," series of exercises that will bring all your major muscles into use easily and painlessly.

There are five graded levels, and as you move from one level to the next, you will be building your body to a practical and satisfying level of fitness. The gradual and progressive approach to physical fitness is a sound approach.

A REASSURING WORD

This program will not make you "muscle-bound." Many women avoid exercise because they are afraid they will become muscle-bound. Actually, little or no exercise does more harm to your muscles, because they lose tone and become less elastic, weaker, and softer. These exercises are designed to firm your muscles, restore their tone, increase their strength and flexibility. Your appearance will improve as certain muscles, in the abdomen and back, for example, become stronger and give you better support. As your arm and leg muscles become firmer, every move you make is likely to be easier and more graceful.

HOW THE PROGRAM WORKS

The program calls for ten mild exercises during the orientation period. Thereafter, you do the warm-up exercises and the seven conditioning exercises listed for each level. The first six exercises of the orientation program are the warm-up exercises. Your daily circulatory exercise is your choice. You can choose: alternate running and walking, skipping rope, running in place. All are effective. On a pleasant day, do the alternate running and walking. When the weather is bad, pick something you can do indoors. And remember, switch around for variety.

HOW YOU PROGRESS

A sound physical-conditioning program should take your personal exercise tolerance into account and allow you to increase your tolerance by increasing your activity gradually. As you move along, you should be doing more and more with less and less exertion. As you move from level to level, some exercises will be modified for increased effort. Others will remain the same, but you will build more strength and stamina by increasing the number of repetitions.

You will be increasing your fitness in another way, too. Level One is designed to reduce the amount of "breathing time" needed between exercises until you can do the seven conditioning exercises without resting. Gradually reducing the time it takes you to do each exercise will benefit your heart and lungs and keep your workouts short. The seven conditioning exercises, however, should not be a race against time. Do each exercise correctly to get the maximum benefit.

CHOOSING YOUR GOAL

This program is designed with a carefully planned progression. There is no need to pick your goal now. Many women will be able to advance through the first three levels. While the fourth is challenging, some women will achieve it. Only vigorous, well-conditioned women, however, will reach the fifth level.

After you complete the early levels of this program, decide if you want to go further. You can go as far as you want. If you exercise daily, you will find you are going even further than you thought possible.

HOW LONG AT EACH LEVEL?

Your objective at each level is to reach the point where you can do all the exercises the number of times indicated without resting. But start slowly. It cannot be emphasized enough that solid fitness is gradual fitness.

The more slowly you build, the less likely you are to strain or pull your muscles.

If you cannot complete any exercise sequence, stop for a brief rest. Then take up where you left off and complete the count. As you move along, though, you will have less difficulty.

Stay at each level for at least three weeks. If you do not pass the prove-out test at the end of that time, stay at that level until you do. The prove-out test calls for doing the seven conditioning exercises three times without stopping and one circulatory activity.

THE TEST: A MEASURE OF YOUR PROGRESS

You will, of course, notice increased strength and stamina from week to week. For one thing, the exercises will become easier. There is also a two-minute step test you can use to measure and keep a running record of your growing strength and stamina. The step test measures your cardiovascular response. Although it does not take long, it is vigorous. Stop if you become overly tired while taking the test. Do not try it until you have completed the orientation period.

Use any sturdy bench or chair 15 to 17 inches in height.

Count 1. Place right foot on bench.

Count 2. Bring left foot alongside of right and stand erect.

Count 3. Lower right foot to floor.

Count 4. Lower left foot to floor.

Repeat the 4-count movement thirty times a minute for two minutes.

Then sit down on bench or chair for two minutes.

Following the 2-minute rest, take your pulse for 30 seconds. Double the count to get the per-minute rate. (You can find the pulse by applying middle and index finger of one hand firmly to the inside of the wrist of the other hand, on the thumb side.)

Record your score for future comparisons. In succeeding tests—about once every two weeks—you will find your pulse rate becoming lower as your physical condition improves.

Three important points:

1. For best results, do not exercise for at least ten minutes before taking the test. Take it at about the same time of day and always use the same bench or chair.
2. Remember that pulse rates vary among individuals. This is an individual test. What is important is not a comparison of your pulse rate with someone else's, but rather a record of how your own rate is reduced as your fitness increases.
3. As you progress, your pulse rate should gradually level off. This is an indication that you are approaching peak fitness.

YOUR PROGRESS RECORDS

Charts are provided for the orientation program and for all five levels.

They list the exercises to be done and the goal for each exercise in terms of number of repetitions, distance, etc.

There is also a space to record your progress—(1) in completing the recommended fifteen workouts at each level, (2) in accomplishing the three prove-out workouts before moving on to a succeeding level, and (3) in the results as you take the step test from time to time.

You do the warm-up exercises and the conditioning exercises along with one circulatory activity for each workout.

Check off each workout as you complete it. The last three numbers are for the prove-out workouts, in which the seven conditioning exercises should be done without resting. Check them off as you accomplish them.

You are now ready for the next level.

Take the step test at two-week intervals and enter your pulse rate.

When you move on to the next level, transfer the last pulse rate from the preceding level. Enter it in the margin to the left of the new progress record and circle it so it will be convenient for continuing reference.

GETTING SET— ORIENTATION WORKOUTS

With the series of ten mild exercises illustrated and described here, you can get yourself ready—without severe aches or pains—for the progressive conditioning program.

Plan on a minimum of one week for preliminary conditioning. Do not hesitate to spend two weeks, or three if necessary, to limber up enough to do all the exercises easily.

1. BEND AND STRETCH

Starting Position: Stand erect, feet shoulder width apart.
Action: Count 1. Bend trunk forward and down, flexing knees. Stretch gently in attempt to touch fingers to toes or floor.
Count 2. Return to starting position.
Note: Do slowly, stretch and relax at intervals rather than in rhythm.

2. KNEE LIFT

Starting Position: Stand erect, feet together, arms at sides.
Action: Count 1. Raise left knee as high as possible, grasping leg with hands and pulling knee against body while keeping back straight.
Count 2. Lower to starting position.
Counts 3 and 4. Repeat with right knee.

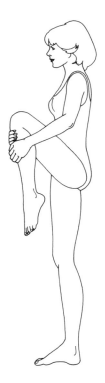

They list the exercises to be done and the goal for each exercise in terms of number of repetitions, distance, etc.

There is also a space to record your progress—(1) in completing the recommended fifteen workouts at each level, (2) in accomplishing the three prove-out workouts before moving on to a succeeding level, and (3) in the results as you take the step test from time to time.

You do the warm-up exercises and the conditioning exercises along with one circulatory activity for each workout.

Check off each workout as you complete it. The last three numbers are for the prove-out workouts, in which the seven conditioning exercises should be done without resting. Check them off as you accomplish them.

You are now ready for the next level.

Take the step test at two-week intervals and enter your pulse rate.

When you move on to the next level, transfer the last pulse rate from the preceding level. Enter it in the margin to the left of the new progress record and circle it so it will be convenient for continuing reference.

GETTING SET— ORIENTATION WORKOUTS

With the series of ten mild exercises illustrated and described here, you can get yourself ready—without severe aches or pains— for the progressive conditioning program.

Plan on a minimum of one week for preliminary conditioning. Do not hesitate to spend two weeks, or three if necessary, to limber up enough to do all the exercises easily.

1. BEND AND STRETCH

Starting Position: Stand erect, feet shoulder width apart.
Action: Count 1. Bend trunk forward and down, flexing knees. Stretch gently in attempt to touch fingers to toes or floor.
Count 2. Return to starting position.
Note: Do slowly, stretch and relax at intervals rather than in rhythm.

2. KNEE LIFT

Starting Position: Stand erect, feet together, arms at sides.
Action: Count 1. Raise left knee as high as possible, grasping leg with hands and pulling knee against body while keeping back straight.
Count 2. Lower to starting position.
Counts 3 and 4. Repeat with right knee.

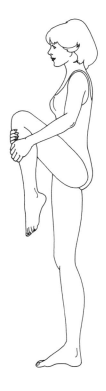

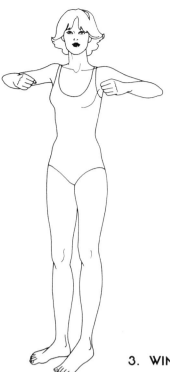

3. WING STRETCHER

Starting Position: Stand erect, elbows at shoulder height, fists clenched in front of chest.

Action: Count 1. Thrust elbows backward vigorously without arching back. Keep head erect, elbows at shoulder height.

Count 2. Return to starting position.

4. HALF KNEE BEND

Starting Position: Stand erect, hands on hips.

Action: Count 1. Bend knees halfway while extending arms forward, palms down.

Count 2. Return to starting position.

Repetitions

Conditioning exercises
*1. Bend and stretch 10
*2. Knee lift .... 10 left, 10 right
*3. Wing stretcher 20
*4. Half knee bend 10
*5. Arm circles .... 15 each way
*6. Body bender .... 10 left, 10 right
 7. Prone arch 10
 8. Knee push-up 6
 9. Head and shoulder curl .. 5
10. Ankle stretch 15

Circulatory activity   Walking .... ½ mile
(choose one   Rope (skip 15 seconds;
each workout)   rest 60 seconds) .... 3 series

* The first six exercises of the orientation program will be used as warm-up exercises throughout the graded levels.
Step Test Record—After completing the orientation program, take the 2-minute step test (as described on page 39). Record your pulse rate here: _____. This will be the base rate with which you can make comparisons in the future.

5. ARM CIRCLES

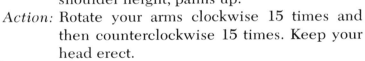

Starting Position: Stand erect, arms extended sideward at shoulder height, palms up.

Action: Rotate your arms clockwise 15 times and then counterclockwise 15 times. Keep your head erect.

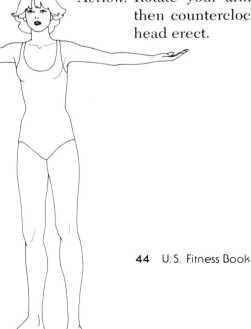

up to sitting position, sliding hands along legs, grasping ankles.

Count 2. Roll back to starting position.

6. LEG RAISER

Starting Position: Right side of body on floor, head resting on right arm.

Action: Lift left leg about 24″ off floor, then lower it. Do required number of repetitions. Repeat on other side.

WOMEN: LEVEL ONE		Goal
Warm-up exercises	Exercises 1–6 of orientation program	
		Uninterrupted repetitions
Conditioning exercises	1. Toe touch	5
	2. Sprinter	8
	3. Sitting stretch	10
	4. Knee push-up	8
	5. Sit-up (arms extended)	5
	6. Leg raiser	5 each leg
	7. Flutter kick	20
Circulatory activity (choose one each workout)	Walking (120 steps a minute)	½ mile
	Rope (skip 30 seconds; rest 60 seconds)	2 series
	Run in place (run 50; straddle hop 10—two cycles)	2 minutes
Water activities	See recommendations in Chapter V.	
Your progress record	1 2 3 4 5 6 7 8 9 10 11 12	13 14 15
Step test (pulse)		Prove-out workouts

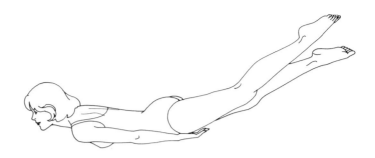

7. FLUTTER KICK

Starting Position: Lie face down, hands tucked under thighs.

Action: Arch the back, bringing chest and head up, then flutter kick continuously, moving the legs 8″–10″ apart. Kick from hips with knees slightly bent. Count each kick as one.

Circulatory Activities

Walking Maintain a pace of 120 steps per minute for a distance of ½ mile. Swing arms and breathe deeply.

Rope Skip or jump rope continuously using any form for 30 seconds and then rest 60 seconds. Repeat 2 times.

Run in Place Raise each foot at least 4″ off the floor and jog in place. Count 1 each time left foot touches floor. Complete number of running steps called for in chart, then do specified number of straddle hops. Complete 2 cycles of alternate running and hopping for time specified on chart.

STRADDLE HOP

Starting Position: At attention.
Action: Count 1. Swing arms sideward and upward, touching hands above head (arms straight) while simultaneously moving feet sideward and apart in a single jumping motion.
Count 2. Spring back to starting position. Two counts in one hop.

WOMEN: LEVEL TWO   1. TOE TOUCH

Starting Position: Stand at attention.
Action: Count 1. Bend trunk forward and down, keeping knees straight, touching fingers to ankles.
Count 2. Bounce and touch fingers to top of feet.
Count 3. Bounce and touch fingers to toes.
Count 4. Return to starting position.

2. SPRINTER

Starting Position: Squat, hands on floor, fingers pointed forward, left leg fully extended to rear.
Action: Count 1. Reverse position of feet in bouncing movement, bringing left foot to hands, extending right leg backward—all in one motion.
Count 2. Reverse feet again, returning to starting position.

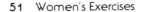

51   Women's Exercises

3. SITTING STRETCH

Starting position: Sit, legs spread apart, hands on knees.
Action: Count 1. Bend forward at waist, extending arms as far forward as possible.
Count 2. Return to starting position.

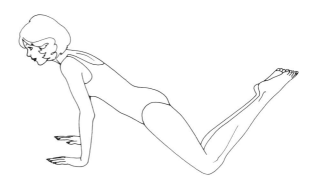

4. KNEE PUSH-UP

Starting Position: Lie on floor, face down, legs together, knees bent with feet raised off floor, hands on floor under shoulders, palms down.
Action: Count 1. Push upper body off floor until arms are fully extended and body is in straight line from head to knees.
Count 2. Return to starting position.

5. SIT-UP (FINGERS LACED)

Starting Position: Lie on back, legs straight and feet spread approximately 1' apart. Fingers laced behind neck.
Action: Count 1. Curl up to sitting position and turn trunk to left. Touch right elbow to left knee.

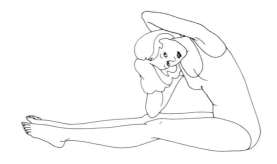

Count 2. Return to starting position.
Count 3. Curl up to sitting position and turn trunk to right. Touch left elbow to right knee.
Count 4. Return to starting position. Score one sit-up each time you return to starting position. Knees may be bent as necessary.

WOMEN: LEVEL TWO												Goal		
Warm-up exercises	Exercises 1–6 of orientation program													
									Uninterrupted repetitions					
Conditioning exercises	1. Toe touch 10													
	2. Sprinter 12													
	3. Sitting stretch 15													
	4. Knee push-up 12													
	5. Sit-up (fingers laced) 10													
	6. Leg raiser .... 10 each leg													
	7. Flutter kick 30													
Circulatory activity (choose one each workout)	Jog-walk (jog 50, walk 50) .... ½ mile													
	Rope (skip 30 seconds; rest 60 seconds) .... 3 series													
	Run in place (run 80, hop 15—two cycles) .... 3 minutes													
Water activities	See recommendations in Chapter V.													
Your progress record	1	2	3	4	5	6	7	8	9	10	11	12	13	14	15
Step test (pulse)													Prove-out workouts		

6. LEG RAISER

Starting Position: Right side of body on floor, head resting on right arm.

Action: Lift left leg about 24″ off floor, then lower it. Do required number of repetitions. Repeat on other side.

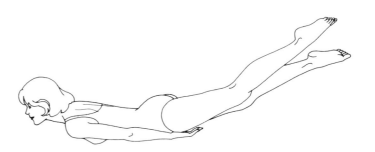

7. FLUTTER KICK

Starting Position: Lie face down, hands tucked under thighs.

Action: Arch the back, bringing chest and head up, then flutter kick continuously, moving the legs 8″–10″ apart. Kick from hips with knees slightly bent. Count each kick as one.

Circulatory Activities

Jog-Walk   Jog and walk alternately for number of paces indicated on chart for distance specified.

Rope   Skip or jump rope continuously using any form for 30 seconds and then rest 60 seconds. Repeat 3 times.

Run in Place Raise each foot at least 4″ off floor and jog in place. Count 1 each time left foot touches floor. Complete number of running steps called for in chart, then do specified number of straddle hops. Complete 2 cycles of alternate running and hopping for time specified on chart.

STRADDLE HOP

Starting Position: At attention.
        Action: Count 1. Swing arms sideward and upward, touching hands above head (arms straight) while simultaneously moving feet sideward and apart in a single jumping motion.
Count 2. Spring back to starting position. Two counts in one hop.

WOMEN: LEVEL THREE   1. TOE TOUCH

Starting Position: Stand at attention.
        Action: Count 1. Bend trunk forward and down, keeping knees straight, touching fingers to ankles.
Count 2. Bounce and touch fingers to top of feet.
Count 3. Bounce and touch fingers to toes.
Count 4. Return to starting position.

2. SPRINTER

Starting Position: Squat, hands on floor, fingers pointed forward, left leg fully extended to rear.

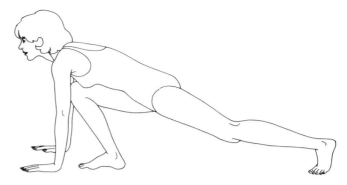

Action: Count 1. Reverse position of feet in bouncing movement, bringing left foot to hands, extending right leg backward—all in one motion.

Count 2. Reverse feet again, returning to starting position.

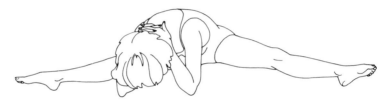

3. SITTING STRETCH (FINGERS LACED)

Starting Position: Sit, legs spread apart, fingers laced behind neck.

Action: Count 1. Bend forward at waist, reaching elbows as close to floor as possible.

Count 2. Return to starting position.

4. KNEE PUSH-UP

Starting Position: Lie on floor, face down, legs together, knees bent with feet raised off floor, hands on floor under shoulders, palms down.

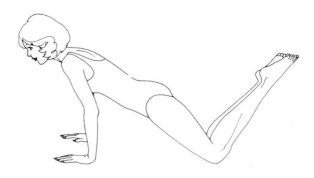

Action: Count 1. Push upper body off floor until arms are fully flexed and body in straight line from head to knees.

Count 2. Return to starting position.

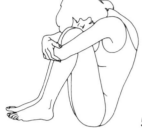

5. SIT-UP (ARMS EXTENDED, KNEES UP)

Starting Position: Lie on back, legs straight, arms extended overhead.

Action: Count 1. Sit up, reaching forward with arms encircling knees while pulling them tightly to chest.

Count 2. Return to starting position. Do this exercise rhythmically, without breaks in the movement.

6. LEG RAISER

Starting Position: Right side of body on floor, head resting on right arm.

Action: Lift left leg about 24" off floor, then lower it. Do required number of repetitions. Repeat on other side.

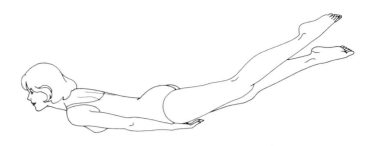

7. FLUTTER KICK

Starting Position: Lie face down, hands tucked under thighs.
Action: Arch the back, bringing chest and head up. Then flutter kick continuously, moving the legs 8″–10″ apart. Kick from hips with knees slightly bent. Count each kick as one.

WOMEN: LEVEL THREE		Goal
Warm-up exercises	Exercises 1–6 of orientation program	
		Uninterrupted repetitions
Conditioning exercises	1. Toe touch	20
	2. Sprinter	16
	3. Sitting stretch (fingers laced) . .	15
	4. Knee push-up	20
	5. Sit-up (arms extended, knees up)	15
	6. Leg raiser	16 each leg
	7. Flutter kick	40
Circulatory activity (choose one each workout)	Jog-walk (jog 50, walk 50)	¾ mile
	Rope (skip 45 seconds; rest 30 seconds)	3 series
	Run in place (run 110, hop 20—two cycles)	4 minutes
Water activities	See recommendations in Chapter V.	

Your progress record	1	2	3	4	5	6	7	8	9	10	11	12	13 14 15
Step test (pulse)													Prove-out workouts

Circulatory Activities

Jog-Walk Jog and walk alternately for number of paces indicated on chart for distance specified.

Rope Skip or jump rope continuously using any form for 45 seconds and then rest 30 seconds. Repeat 3 times.

Run in Place Raise each foot at least 4″ off floor and jog in place. Count 1 each time left foot touches floor. Complete number of running steps called for in chart, then do specified number of straddle hops. Complete 2 cycles of alternate running and hopping for time specified on chart.

STRADDLE HOP

Starting Position: At attention.
Action: Count 1. Swing arms sideward and upward, touching hands above head (arms straight) while simultaneously moving feet sideward and apart in a single jumping motion.
Count 2. Spring back to starting position. Two counts in one hop.

WOMEN: LEVEL FOUR   1. TOE TOUCH (TWIST AND BEND)

Starting Position: Stand, feet shoulder width apart, arms extended overhead, thumbs interlocked.

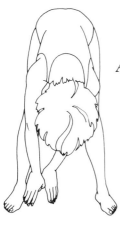

Action: Count 1. Twist trunk to right and touch floor inside right foot with fingers of both hands.
Count 2. Touch floor outside toes of right foot.
Count 3. Touch floor outside heel of right foot.
Count 4. Return to starting position, sweeping trunk and arms upward in a wide arc. On the next four counts, repeat action to left side.

2. SPRINTER

Starting Position: Squat, hands on floor, fingers pointed forward, left leg fully extended to rear.
Action: Count 1. Reverse position of feet in bouncing movement, bringing left foot to hands, extending right leg backward—all in one motion.
Count 2. Reverse feet again, returning to starting position.

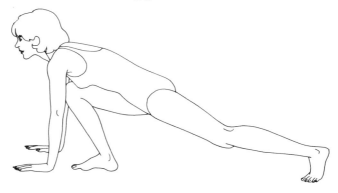

3. SITTING STRETCH (ALTERNATE)

Starting Position: Sit, legs spread apart, fingers laced behind neck, elbows back.

Action: Count 1. Bend forward to left, touching forehead to left knee.

Count 2. Return to starting position.

Counts 3 and 4. Repeat to right. Score one repetition each time you return to starting position. Knees may be bent if necessary.

4. PUSH-UP

Starting Position: Lie on floor, face down, legs together, hands on floor under shoulders with fingers pointing straight ahead.

Action: Count 1. Push body off floor by extending arms so that weight rests on hands and toes.

Count 2. Lower the body until chest touches floor.

Note: Body should be kept straight, buttocks should not be raised, abdomen should not sag.

5. SIT-UP (ARMS CROSSED, KNEES BENT)

Starting Position: Lie on back, arms crossed on chest, hands grasping opposite shoulders, knees bent to right angle, feet flat on floor.

Action: Count 1. Curl up to sitting position.

Count 2. Return to starting position.

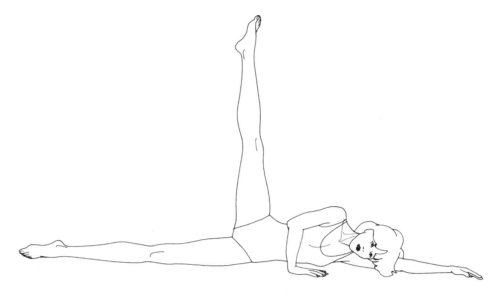

6. LEG RAISER (WHIP)

Starting Position: Right side of body on floor, right arm supporting head.

Action: Whip left leg up and down rapidly lifting as high as possible off the floor. Count each whip as one. Reverse position and whip right leg up and down.

7. PRONE ARCH (ARMS EXTENDED)

Starting Position: Lie face down, legs straight and together, arms extended to sides at shoulder level.

Action: Count 1. Arch the back, bringing arms, chest and head up, and raising legs as high as possible.

Count 2. Return to starting position.

		Uninterrupted repetitions
Warm-up exercises	Exercises 1–6 of orientation program	
Conditioning exercises	1. Toe touch (twist and bend)	
	2. Sprinter	15 each side
	3. Sitting stretch (alternate)	20
	4. Push-up	20
	5. Sit-up (arms crossed, knees bent)	8 20
	6. Leg raiser (whip)	10 each leg
	7. Prone arch (arms extended)	15
Circulatory activity (choose one each workout)	Jog-walk (jog 100; walk 50)	1 mile
	Rope (skip 60 seconds; rest 30 seconds)	3 series
	Run in place (run 145, hop 25—two cycles)	5 minutes
Water activities	See recommendations in Chapter V.	

	1	2	3	4	5	6	7	8	9	10	11	12	13	14	15
Your progress record													Prove-out workouts		
Step test (pulse)															

Circulatory Activities

Jog-Walk   Jog and walk alternately for number of paces indicated on chart for distance specified.

Rope   Skip or jump rope continuously using any form for 60 seconds and then rest 30 seconds. Repeat 3 times.

Run in Place   Raise each foot at least 4″ off floor and jog in place. Count 1 each time left foot touches floor. Complete number of running steps called for in chart, then do specified number of straddle hops. Complete 2 cycles of alternate running and hopping for time specified on chart.

STRADDLE HOP

Starting Position: At attention.
Action: Count 1. Swing arms sideward and upward, touching hands above head (arms straight) while simultaneously moving feet sideward and apart in a single jumping motion.
Count 2. Spring back to starting position. Two counts in one hop.

WOMEN: LEVEL FIVE   **1. TOE TOUCH (TWIST AND BEND)**

Starting Position: Stand, feet shoulder width apart, arms extended overhead, thumbs interlocked.
Action: Count 1. Twist trunk to right and touch floor inside right foot with fingers of both hands.
Count 2. Touch floor outside toes of right foot.
Count 3. Touch floor outside heel of right foot.
Count 4. Return to starting position, sweeping trunk and arms upward in a wide arc. On the next four counts, repeat action to left side.

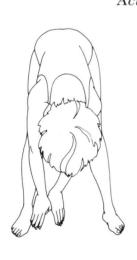

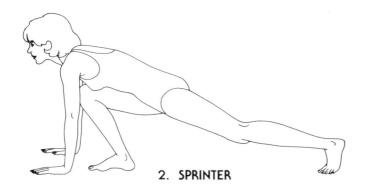

2. SPRINTER

Starting Position: Squat, hands on floor, fingers pointed forward, left leg fully extended to rear.

Action: Count 1. Reverse position of feet in bouncing movement, bringing left foot to hands
and extending right leg backward—all in
one motion.

Count 2. Reverse feet again, returning to
starting position.

3. SITTING STRETCH (ALTERNATE)

Starting Position: Sit, legs spread apart, fingers behind neck,
elbows back.

Action: Count 1. Bend forward to left, touching forehead to left knee.

Count 2. Return to starting position.

Counts 3 and 4. Repeat to right. Score one
repetition each time you return to starting
position. Knees may be bent if necessary.

4. PUSH-UP

Starting Position: Lie on floor, face down, legs together, hands
on floor under shoulders with fingers point-
ing straight ahead.

Action: Count 1. Push body off floor by extending arms so that weight rests on hands and toes. Count 2. Lower the body until chest touches floor.

Note: Body should be kept straight, buttocks should not be raised, abdomen should not sag.

5. SIT-UP (FINGERS LACED, KNEES BENT)

Starting Postion: Lie on back, fingers laced behind neck, knees bent, feet flat on floor.

Action: Count 1. Sit up, turn trunk to right, touch left elbow to right knee.

Count 2. Return to starting position.

Count 3. Sit up, turn trunk to left, touch right elbow to left knee.

Count 4. Return to starting position. Score one each time you return to starting position.

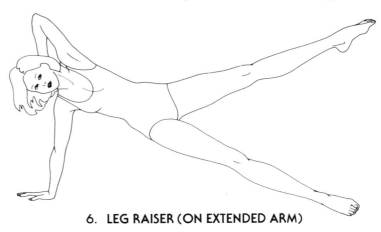

6. LEG RAISER (ON EXTENDED ARM)

Starting Position: Body rigidly supported by extended right arm and foot. Left arm is held behind head

Action: Count 1. Raise left leg high.

Count 2. Return to starting position slowly.
Repeat on other side. Do required number
of repetitions.

7. PRONE ARCH (FINGERS LACED)

Starting Position: Lie face down, fingers laced behind neck.

Action: Count 1. Arch back, legs and chest off floor.

Count 2. Extend arms fully forward.

Count 3. Return hands to behind neck.

Count 4. Flatten body to floor.

WOMEN: LEVEL FIVE	Goal
Warm-up exercises	Exercises 1–6 of orientation program
	Uninterrupted repetitions
Conditioning exercises	1. Toe touch (twist and bend) . . . . 25 each side
	2. Sprinter 24
	3. Sitting stretch (alternate) 26
	4. Push-up 15
	5. Sit-up (fingers laced, knees bent) 25
	6. Leg raiser (on extended arm) . . 10 each side
	7. Prone arch (fingers laced) 25
Circulatory activity (choose one each workout)	Jog-run . . . . 1 mile
	Rope (skip 2 minutes; rest 45 seconds) . . . . 2 series
	Run in place (run 180, hop 30—two cycles) . . . . 6 minutes
Water activities	See recommendations in Chapter V.
Your progress record	1 2 3 4 5 6 7 8 9 10 11 12 │ 13 14 15
Step test (pulse)	│ Prove-out workouts

Circulatory Activities

Jog-Run Jog and run alternately for distance specified on chart.

Rope Skip or jump rope continuously using any form for 2 minutes and then rest 45 seconds. Repeat 2 times.

Run in Place Raise each foot at least 4" off floor and jog in place. Count 1 each time left foot touches floor. Complete number of running steps called for in chart, then do specified number of straddle hops. Complete 2 cycles of alternate running and hopping in time specified on the chart.

STRADDLE HOP

Starting Position: At attention.
Action: Count 1. Swing arms sideward and upward, touching hands above head (arms straight) while simultaneously moving feet sideward and apart in a single jumping motion.
Count 2. Spring back to starting position. Two counts in one hop.

STAYING FIT

Once you have reached the level of fitness you have chosen for yourself, you will want to maintain your level.

To do so, work out daily at that level.

While it has been found possible to maintain fitness with three workouts a week, ideally, exercise should be a daily habit. If you can, by all means continue your workouts on a five-times-a-week basis.

If at any point while reaching for or maintaining your goal, the workouts are interrupted for more than a week, begin again at a lower level. If you have had a serious illness or surgery, check with your physician before you begin again.

BROADENING YOUR PROGRAM

The exercises and activities you have been doing are basic. They are designed only to take you soundly and progressively to physical fitness without need for special equipment or facilities.

There are many other activities and forms of exercise which you may use to supplement the basic program. You will find them discussed in Chapter V.

They include a variety of sports; water exercises (if you have access to a pool); and isometrics (sometimes called exercises without movement) which take little time (6–8 seconds each). One isometric, the abdominal, is particularly valuable for many women; it helps strengthen muscles that can act like a girdle to maintain a trim waistline.

You will find suggestions, too, for improving your posture and for taking advantage of many daily opportunities for sound physical activity.

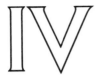

Men's Exercises

This program is designed for the man who has not done any consistent, vigorous, all-around exercise recently. Playing golf once a week, or tennis once a month, does not fit this definition. The program starts with an orientation, or "get-set," series of exercises that will bring all your major muscles into use easily and painlessly.

There are then five graded levels, and as you move from one level to the next, you will be building your body to a practical and satisfying level of fitness. The gradual and progressive approach to physical fitness is a sound approach.

HOW THE PROGRAM WORKS

The program calls for ten mild exercises during the orientation period. Thereafter, you do the warm-up exercises and the seven conditioning exercises listed for each level. The first six exercises of the orientation program are the warm-up exercises. Your daily circulatory exercise is your choice. You can choose: alternate running and walking, skipping rope, running in place. All are effective. On a pleasant day, do the alternate running and walking. When the weather is bad, pick something you can do indoors. And remember, switch around for variety.

HOW YOU PROGRESS

Right now, you probably have a limited tolerance for exercise. You can do just so much without becoming tired. A sound physical conditioning program should take your personal exercise tolerance into account. A sound program should also allow you to increase your tolerance by increasing your activity gradually. As you move along, you should be doing more and more with less and less exertion. As you move from level to level, some exercises will be modified for increased effort. Others will remain the same, but you will build more strength and stamina by increasing the number of repetitions.

You will be increasing your fitness another way, too. Level One is designed to reduce the amount of "breathing time" needed between exercises until you can do the seven conditioning exercises without resting. Gradually reducing the time it takes you to do each exercise will benefit your heart and lungs and keep your workouts short. The seven conditioning exercises, however should not be a race against time. Do each exercise correctly to get the maximum benefit.

CHOOSING YOUR GOAL

This program is designed with a carefully planned progression. There is no need to pick your goal now. Many men will be able to advance through the first three levels. While the fourth is challenging, some men will achieve it. Only vigorous, well-conditioned men, however, will reach the fifth level. If you do not reach the last level, do not be discouraged. Not everybody is physically constituted to play par golf or run a mile in under four minutes. Your peak level also depends on your age, previous conditioning, and your determination.

Chances are that, after several months of workouts, you will be surprised at how much you can do. As your physical tolerance for exercise increases, so will your psychological tolerance. As you progress, you may realize that you can and want to go a long way. Go as far as you like.

HOW LONG AT EACH LEVEL?

Your objective at each level is to reach the point where you can do all the exercises the number of times indicated without resting. But start slowly. It cannot be emphasized enough: solid fitness is gradual fitness. The more slowly you build, the less likely you are to strain or pull your muscles.

If you cannot complete any exercise sequence, stop for a brief rest. Then take up where you left off and complete the count. As you move along, though, you will have less difficulty.

Stay at each level for at least three weeks. If you do not pass the prove-out test at the end of that time, stay at that level until you do. The prove-out test calls for doing the seven conditioning exercises three times without stopping and one circulatory activity.

THE TEST: A MEASURE OF YOUR PROGRESS

You will, of course, notice increased strength and stamina from week to week. For one thing, the exercises will become easier. There is also a two-minute step test you can use to measure and keep a running record of your growing strength and stamina. The step test measures your cardiovascular response. Although it does not take long, it is vigorous. Stop if you become overly tired while taking the test. Do not try it until you have completed the orientation period.

Use any sturdy bench or chair 15–17 inches in height.

Count 1. Place right foot on bench.

Count 2. Bring left foot alongside of right and stand erect.

Count 3. Lower right foot to floor.

Count 4. Lower left foot to floor.

Repeat the 4-count movement 30 times a minute for two minutes.

Then sit down on bench or chair for two minutes.

Following the 2-minute rest, take your pulse for 30 seconds. Double the count to get the per-minute rate. (You can find the pulse by applying middle and index fingers of one hand firmly to the inside of the wrist of the other hand, on the thumb side.)

Record your score for future comparisons. In succeeding tests—about once every two weeks—you probably will find your pulse rate becoming lower as your physical condition improves.

Three important points:

1. For best results, do not exercise for at least ten minutes before taking the test. Take it at about the same time of day and always use the same bench or chair.
2. Remember that pulse rates vary among individuals. This is an individual test. What is important is not a comparison of your pulse rate with someone else's —but rather a record of how your own rate is reduced as your fitness increases.
3. As you progress, the rate at which your pulse rate is lowered should gradually level off. This is an indication that you are approaching peak fitness.

YOUR PROGRESS RECORDS

Charts are provided for the orientation program and for all five levels.

They list the exercises to be done and the goal for each exercise in terms of number of repetitions, distance, etc.

There is a space in which to record your progress—(1) in completing the recommended 15 workouts at each level, (2) in accomplishing the three prove-out workouts before moving on to a succeeding level, and (3) in the results as you take the step test from time to time.

You do the warm-up exercises and the conditioning exercises along with one circulatory activity for each workout.

Check off each workout as you complete it. The last three numbers are for the proveout workouts, in which the seven conditioning exercises should be done without resting. Check them off as you accomplish them.

You are now ready for the next level.

Take the step test at about 2-week intervals and enter your pulse rate.

When you move on to the next level, transfer the last pulse rate from the preceding level. Enter it in the margin to the left of the new progress record and circle it so it will be convenient for continuing reference.

GETTING SET—ORIENTATION WORKOUTS

With the series of preliminary exercises listed in the chart on page 77 and illustrated and described on the following pages, you can get yourself ready, without severe aches or pains, for the progressive conditioning program.

Even if these preliminary exercises seem easy—and they are meant to be mild—plan on a minimum of one week with them. Do not hesitate to spend two weeks or even three if necessary for you to limber up enough so you can accomplish all the exercises easily.

1. BEND AND STRETCH

Starting Position: Stand erect, feet shoulder width apart.

Action: Count 1. Bend trunk forward and down, flexing knees. Stretch gently in attempt to touch
fingers to toes or floor.
Count 2. Return to starting position.
Note: Do slowly, stretch and relax at intervals rather than in rhythm.

2. KNEE LIFT

Starting Position: Stand erect feet together, arms at sides.
Action: Count 1. Raise left knee as high as possible,
grasping leg with hands and pulling knee
against body while keeping back straight.
Count 2. Lower to starting position.
Counts 3 and 4. Repeat with right knee.

3. WING STRETCHER

Starting Position: Stand erect, elbows at shoulder height, fists
clenched in front of chest.
Action: Count 1. Thrust elbows backward vigorously without arching back. Keep head erect,
elbows at shoulder height.
Count 2. Return to starting position.

4. HALF KNEE BEND

Starting Position: Stand erect, hands on hips.
Action: Count 1. Bend knees halfway while extend-
ing arms forward, palms down.
Count 2. Return to starting position.

		Repetitions
Conditioning exercises	*1. Bend and stretch	10
	*2. Knee lift	10 left, 10 right
	*3. Wing stretcher	20
	*4. Half knee bend	10
	*5. Arm circles	15 each way
	*6. Body bender	10 left, 10 right
	7. Prone arch	10
	8. Knee push-up	6
	9. Head and shoulder curl . .	5
	10. Ankle stretch	15
Circulatory activity	Walking	½ mile
(choose one	Rope (skip 15 seconds;	
each workout)	rest 60 seconds)	3 series

* The first six exercises of the orientation program will be used as warm-up exercises throughout the graded levels.
Step Test Record—After completing the orientation program, take the 2-minute step test (as described on page 73). Record your pulse rate here: _____. This will be the base rate with which you can make comparisons in the future.

5. ARM CIRCLES

Starting Position: Stand erect, arms extended sideward at shoulder height, palms up.

Action: Rotate your arms clockwise 15 times and then counterclockwise 15 times. Keep your head erect.

6. BODY BENDER

Starting Position: Stand, feet shoulder width apart, hands behind neck, fingers interlaced.

Action: Count 1. Bend trunk sideward to left as far as possible, keeping hands behind neck.
Count 2. Return to starting position.
Counts 3 and 4. Repeat to the right.

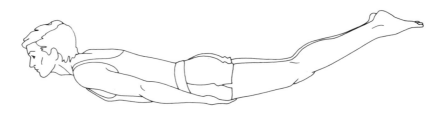

7. PRONE ARCH

Starting Position: Lie face down, hands tucked under thighs.
Action: Count 1. Raise head, shoulders, and legs from floor.
Count 2. Return to starting position.

8. KNEE PUSH-UP

Starting Position: Lie on floor, face down, legs together, knees bent with feet raised off floor.
Action: Count 1. Push upper body off floor until arms are fully extended and body is in straight line from head to knees.
Count 2. Return to starting position.

9. HEAD AND SHOULDER CURL

Starting Position: Lie on back, hands tucked under small of back, palms down.
Action: Count 1. Tighten abdominal muscles, lift head and pull shoulders and elbows up off floor. Hold for four seconds.
Count 2. Return to starting position.

10. ANKLE STRETCH

Starting Position: Stand on a stair, large book or block of wood, with weight on balls of feet and heels raised.
Action: Count 1. Lower heels.
Count 2. Raise heels.

Circulatory Activities

Walking   Step off at a lively pace, swing arms and breathe deeply.

Rope   Any form of skipping or jumping is acceptable. Gradually increase the tempo as your skill and condition improve.

MEN: LEVEL ONE   **1. TOE TOUCH**

Starting Position: Stand at attention.
Action: Count 1. Bend trunk forward and down keeping knees straight, touching fingers to ankles.
Count 2. Bounce and touch fingers to top of feet.
Count 3. Bounce and touch fingers to toes.
Count 4. Return to starting position.

2. SPRINTER

Starting Position: Squat, hands on floor, fingers pointed forward, left leg fully extended to rear.

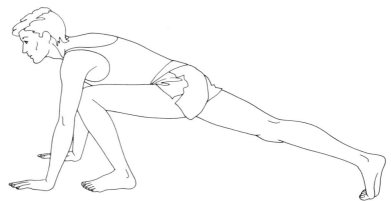

Action: Count 1. Reverse position of feet in bouncing movement, bringing left foot to hands and extending right leg backward—all in one motion.

Count 2. Reverse feet again, returning to starting position.

3. SITTING STRETCH

Starting Position: Sit, legs spread apart, hands on knees.
Action: Count 1. Bend forward at waist, extending arms as far forward as possible.

Count 2. Return to starting position.

4. PUSH-UP

Starting Position: Lie on floor, face down, legs together, hands on floor under shoulders with fingers pointing straight ahead.
Action: Count 1. Push body off floor by extending arms, so that weight rests on hands and toes.

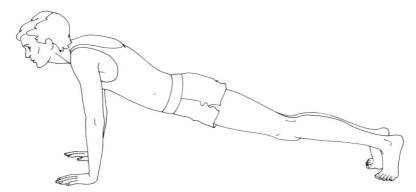

Count 2. Lower the body until chest touches floor.

Note: Body should be kept straight, buttocks should not be raised, abdomen should not sag.

5. SIT-UP (ARMS EXTENDED)

Starting Position: Lie on back, legs straight and together, arms extended beyond head.

Action: Count 1. Bring arms forward over head, roll up to sitting position, sliding hands along legs, grasping ankles.

Count 2. Roll back to starting position.

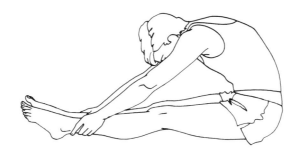

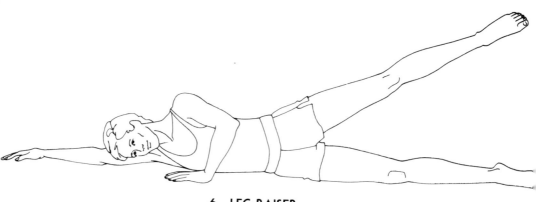

6. LEG RAISER

Starting Position: Right side of body on floor, head resting on right arm.

Action: Lift left leg about 24″ off floor, then lower it. Do required number of repetitions. Repeat on other side.

MEN: LEVEL ONE		Goal
Warm-up exercises	Exercises 1–6 of orientation program	
Conditioning exercises		Uninterrupted repetitions
	1. Toe touch	10
	2. Sprinter	12
	3. Sitting stretch	12
	4. Push-up	4
	5. Sit-up (arms extended)	5
	6. Leg raiser	12 each leg
	7. Flutter kick	30
Circulatory activity (choose one each workout)	Walking (120 steps a minute)	1 mile
	Rope (skip 30 seconds; rest 30 seconds)	2 series
	Run in place (run 60, hop 10—two cycles)	2 minutes
Water activities	See recommendations in Chapter V.	

Your progress record	1	2	3	4	5	6	7	8	9	10	11	12	13	14	15
Step test (pulse)													Prove-out workouts		

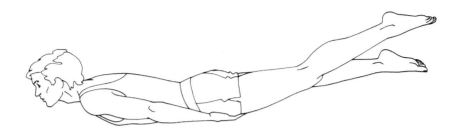

7. FLUTTER KICK

Starting Position: Lie face down, hands tucked under thighs.
Action: Arch the back, bringing chest and head up, then flutter kick continuously, moving the legs 8"–10" apart. Kick from hips with knees slightly bent. Count each kick as one.

Circulatory Activities

Walking Maintain a pace of 120 steps per minute for a distance of 1 mile. Swing arms and breathe deeply.

Rope Skip or jump rope continuously using any form for 30 seconds and then rest 30 seconds. Repeat 2 times.

Run in Place Raise each foot at least 4" off floor and jog in place. Count 1 each time left foot touches floor. Complete the number of running steps called for in chart, then do specified number of straddle hops. Complete 2 cycles of alternate running and hopping for time specified on chart.

STRADDLE HOP

Starting Position: At attention.
       Action: Count 1. Swing arms sideward and upward, touching hands above head (arms straight) while simultaneously moving feet sideward and apart in a single jumping motion.
Count 2. Spring back to starting position. Two counts in one hop.

MEN: LEVEL TWO   1. TOE TOUCH

Starting Position: Stand at attention.
       Action: Count 1. Bend trunk forward and down keeping knees straight, touching fingers to ankles.
Count 2. Bounce and touch fingers to top of feet.
Count 3. Bounce and touch fingers to toes.
Count 4. Return to starting position.

2. SPRINTER

Starting Position: Squat, hands on floor, fingers pointed forward, left leg fully extended to rear.

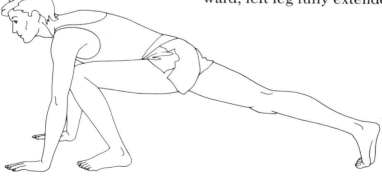

Action: Count 1. Reverse position of feet in bouncing movement, bringing left foot to hands and extending right leg backward—all in one motion.

Count 2. Reverse feet again, returning to starting position

3. SITTING STRETCH

Starting Position: Sit, legs spread apart, hands on knees.
Action: Count 1. Bend forward at waist, extending arms as far forward as possible.
Count 2. Return to starting position.

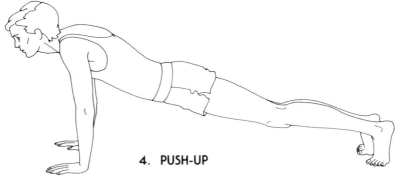

4. PUSH-UP

Starting Position: Lie on floor, face down, legs together, hands on floor under shoulders with fingers pointing straight ahead.
Action: Count 1. Push body off floor by extending arms, so that weight rests on hands and toes.
Count 2. Lower the body until chest touches floor.
Note: Body should be kept straight, buttocks should not be raised, abdomen should not sag.

5. SIT-UP (FINGERS LACED)

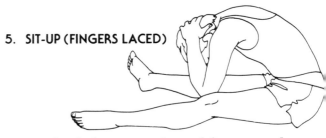

Starting Position: Lie on back, legs straight and feet spread approximately 1' apart. Fingers laced behind neck.

Action: Count 1. Curl up to sitting position and turn trunk to left. Touch the right elbow to left knee.

Count 2. Return to starting position.

Count 3. Curl up to sitting position and turn trunk to right. Touch left elbow to right knee.

Count 4. Return to starting position. Score one situp each time you return to starting position. Knees may be bent as necessary.

6. LEG RAISER

Starting Position: Right side of body on floor, head resting on right arm.

Action: Lift left leg about 24" off floor, then lower it. Do required number of repetitions. Repeat on other side.

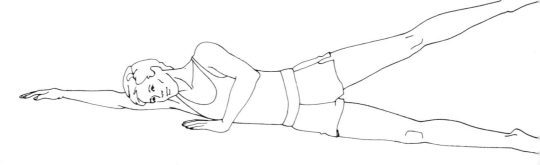

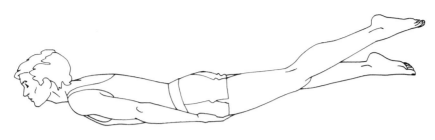

7. FLUTTER KICK

Starting Position: Lie face down, hands tucked under thighs.

Action: Arch the back, bringing chest and head up, then flutter kick continuously, moving the legs 8"–10" apart. Kick from hips with knees slightly bent. Count each kick as one.

	MEN: LEVEL TWO	Goal
Warm-up exercises	Exercises 1–6 of orientation program	
		Uninterrupted repetitions
Conditioning exercises	1. Toe touch	20
	2. Sprinter	16
	3. Sitting stretch	18
	4. Push-up	10
	5. Sit-up (fingers laced)	20
	6. Leg raiser	16 each leg
	7. Flutter kick	40
Circulatory activity (choose one each workout)	Jog-walk (jog 100; walk 100)	1 mile
	Rope (skip 1 minute; rest 1 minute	3 series
	Run in place (run 95, hop 15—two cycles)	3 minutes
Water activities	See recommendations in Chapter V.	
Your progress record	1 2 3 4 5 6 7 8 9 10 11 12	13 14 15
Step test (pulse)		Prove-out workouts

Circulatory Activities

Jog-Walk Jog and walk alternately for number of paces indicated on chart for distance specified.

Rope Skip or jump rope continuously using any form for 60 seconds and then rest 60 seconds. Repeat 3 times.

Run in Place Raise each foot at least 4" off floor and jog in place. Count 1 each time left foot touches floor. Complete the number of running steps called for in chart, then do specified number of straddle hops. Complete 2 cycles of alternate running and hopping for time specified on chart.

STRADDLE HOP

Starting Position: At attention.
Action: Count 1. Swing arms sideward and upward, touching hands above head (arms straight) while simultaneously moving feet sideward and apart in a single jumping motion.
Count 2. Spring back to starting position. Two counts in one hop.

MEN: LEVEL THREE   1. TOE TOUCH

Starting Position: Stand at attention.
Action: Count 1. Bend trunk forward and down

keeping knees straight, touching fingers to ankles.

Count 2. Bounce and touch fingers to top of feet.

Count 3. Bounce and touch fingers to toes.

Count 4. Return to starting position.

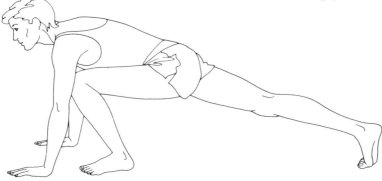

2. SPRINTER

Starting Position: Squat, hands on floor, fingers pointed forward, left leg fully extended to rear.

Action: Count 1. Reverse position of feet in bouncing movement, bringing left foot to hands, extending right leg backward—all in one motion.

Count 2. Reverse feet again, returning to starting position.

3. SITTING STRETCH (FINGERS LACED)

Starting Position: Sit, legs spread apart, fingers laced behind neck, elbows back.

Action: Count 1. Bend forward at waist, reaching elbows as close to floor as possible.

Count 2. Return to starting position.

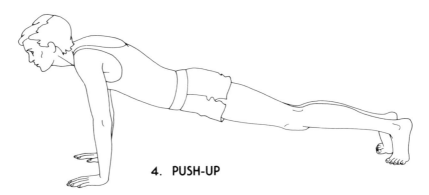

4. PUSH-UP

Starting Position: Lie on floor, face down, legs together, hands on floor under shoulders with fingers pointing straight ahead.

Action: Count 1. Push body off floor by extending arms, so that weight rests on hands and toes. Count 2. Lower the body until chest touches floor.

Note: Body should be kept straight, buttocks should not be raised, abdomen should not sag.

5. SIT-UP (ARMS EXTENDED, KNEES UP)

Starting Position: Lie on back, legs straight, arms extended overhead.

Action: Count 1. Sit up, reaching forward with arms encircling knees while pulling them tightly to chest.

Count 2. Return to starting position. Do this exercise rhythmically, without breaks in the movement.

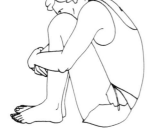

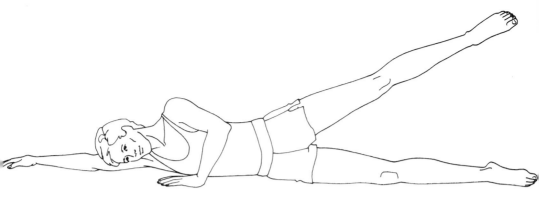

6. LEG RAISER

Starting Position: Right side of body on floor, head resting on right arm.

Action: Lift left leg about 24″ off floor then lower it. Do required number of repetitions. Repeat on other side.

MEN: LEVEL THREE		Goal
Warm-up exercises	Exercises 1–6 of orientation program	
		Uninterrupted repetitions
Conditioning exercises	1. Toe touch	
	2. Sprinter	30
	3. Sitting stretch (fingers laced) . .	20
	4. Push-up	18
	5. Sit-up (arms extended, knees	20
	up)	30
	6. Leg raiser	20 each leg
	7. Flutter kick	50
Circulatory activity (choose one each workout)	Jog-walk (jog 200; walk 100)	1½ miles
	Rope (skip 1 minute; rest 1 minute)	5 series
	Run in place (run 135, hop 20—two cycles)	4 minutes
Water activities	See recommendations in Chapter V.	
Your progress record	1 2 3 4 5 6 7 8 9 10 11 12	13 14 15
Step test (pulse)		Prove-out workouts

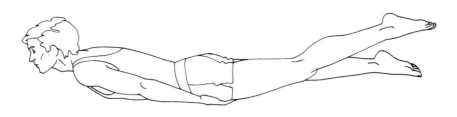

7. FLUTTER KICK

Starting Position: Lie face down, hands tucked under thighs.
Action: Arch the back, bringing chest and head up, then flutter kick continuously, moving the legs 8″–10″ apart. Kick from hips with knees slightly bent. Count each kick as one.

Circulatory Activities

Jog-Walk   Jog and walk alternately for number of paces indicated on chart for distance specified.

Rope   Skip or jump rope continuously using any form for 60 seconds and then rest 60 seconds. Repeat 5 times.

Run in Place   Raise each foot at least 4″ off floor and jog in place. Count 1 each time left foot touches floor. Complete number of running steps called for in chart, then do specified number of straddle hops. Complete 2 cycles of alternate running and hopping for time specified on chart.

STRADDLE HOP

Starting Position: At attention.
Action: Count 1. Swing arms sideward and upward,

touching hands above head (arms straight) while simultaneously moving feet sideward and apart in a single jumping motion.

Count 2. Spring back to starting position. Two counts in one hop.

MEN: LEVEL FOUR

1. TOE TOUCH (TWIST AND BEND)

Starting Position: Stand, feet shoulder width apart, arms extended over head, thumbs interlocked.

Action: Count 1. Twist trunk to right and touch floor inside right foot with fingers of both hands.

Count 2. Touch floor outside toes of right foot.

Count 3. Touch floor outside heel of right foot.

Count 4. Return to starting position, sweeping trunk and arms upward in a wide arc. On the next four counts, repeat action to left side.

2. SPRINTER

Starting Position: Squat, hands on floor, fingers pointed forward, left leg fully extended to rear.

Action: Count 1. Reverse position of feet in bouncing movement, bringing left foot to hands, extending right leg backward—all in one motion.

Count 2. Reverse feet again, returning to starting position.

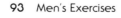

93   Men's Exercises

3. SITTING STRETCH (ALTERNATE)

Starting Position: Sit, legs spread apart, fingers laced behind neck, elbows back.

Action: Count 1. Bend forward to left, touching forehead to left knee.

Count 2. Return to starting position.

Counts 3 and 4. Repeat to right. Score one repetition each time you return to starting position. Knees may be bent if necessary.

4. PUSH-UP

Starting Position: Lie on floor, face down, legs together, hands on floor under shoulders with fingers pointing straight ahead.

Action: Count 1. Push body off floor by extending arms, so that weight rests on hands and toes.

Count 2. Lower the body until chest touches floor.

Note: Body should be kept straight, buttocks should not be raised, abdomen should not sag.

5. SIT-UP (ARMS CROSSED, KNEES BENT)

Starting Position: Lie on back, arms crossed on chest, hands grasping opposite shoulders, knees bent to right angle, feet flat on floor.

Action: Count 1. Curl up to sitting position.
Count 2. Return to starting position.

6. LEG RAISER (WHIP)

Starting Position: Right side of body on floor, right arm supporting head.
Action: Whip left leg up and down rapidly, lifting as high as possible off the floor. Count each whip as one. Reverse position and whip right leg up and down.

MEN: LEVEL FOUR												Goal		
Warm-up exercises	Exercises 1–6 of orientation program													
	Uninterrupted repetitions													
Conditioning exercises	1. Toe touch (twist and bend)													
	2. Sprinter										20 each side			
	3. Sitting stretch (alternate)										28			
	4. Push-up										24			
	5. Sit-up (arms crossed, knees bent)										30 30			
	6. Leg raiser (whip)										20 each leg			
	7. Prone arch (arms extended										20			
Circulatory activity (choose one each workout)	Jog										1 mile			
	Rope (skip 90 seconds; rest 30 seconds)										3 series			
	Run in place (run 180; hop 25—two cycles)										5 minutes			
Water activities	See recommendations in Chapter V.													
Your progress record	1	2	3	4	5	6	7	8	9	10	11	12	13 14 15	
Step test (pulse)													Prove-out workouts	

7. PRONE ARCH (ARMS EXTENDED)

Starting Position: Lie face down, legs straight and together, arms extended to sides at shoulder level.

Action: Count 1. Arch the back, bringing arms, chest and head up, and raising legs as high as possible.

Count 2. Return to starting position.

Circulatory Activities

Jog   Jog continuously for 1 mile.

Rope   Skip or jump rope continuously using any form for 90 seconds and then rest for 30 seconds. Repeat 3 times.

Run in Place   Raise each foot at least 4" off floor and jog in place. Count 1 each time left foot touches floor. Complete number of running steps called for in chart, then do specified number of straddle hops. Complete 2 cycles of alternate running and hopping in time specified on chart.

STRADDLE HOP

Starting Position: At attention.

Action: Count 1. Swing arms sideward and upward, touching hands above head (arms straight) while simultaneously moving feet sideward and apart in a single jumping motion.

Count 2. Spring back to starting position. Two counts in one hop.

1. TOE TOUCH (TWIST AND BEND)

Starting Position: Stand, feet shoulder width apart, arms extended over head, thumbs interlocked.

Action: Count 1. Twist trunk to right and touch floor inside right foot with fingers of both hands.

Count 2. Touch floor outside toes of right foot.

Count 3. Touch floor outside heel of right foot.

Count 4. Return to starting position, sweeping trunk and arms upward in a wide arc. On the next four counts, repeat action to left side.

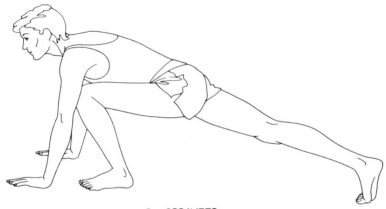

2. SPRINTER

Starting Position: Squat, hands on floor, fingers pointed forward, left leg fully extended to rear.

Action: Count 1. Reverse position of feet in bouncing movement, bringing left foot to hands and extending right leg backward—all in one motion.

Count 2. Reverse feet again, returning to starting position.

97   Men's Exercises

3. SITTING STRETCH (ALTERNATE)

Starting Position: Sit, legs spread apart, fingers laced behind neck, elbows back.

Action: Count 1. Bend forward to left, touching forehead to left knee.

Count 2. Return to starting position.

Counts 3 and 4. Repeat to right. Score one repetition each time you return to starting position. Knees may be bent if necessary.

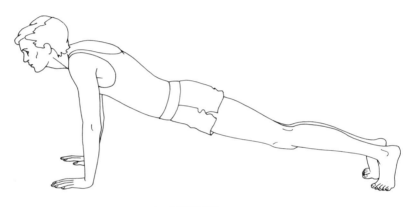

4. PUSH-UP

Starting Position: Lie on floor, face down, legs together, hands on floor under shoulders with fingers pointing straight ahead.

Action: Count 1. Push body off floor by extending arms so that weight rests on hands and toes.

Count 2. Lower body until chest touches floor.

Note: Body should be kept straight, buttocks should not be raised, abdomen should not sag.

5. SIT-UP (FINGERS LACED, KNEES BENT)

Starting Position: Lie on back, fingers laced behind neck, knees bent, feet flat on floor.

Action: Count 1. Sit up, turn trunk to right, touch left elbow to right knee.

Count 2. Return to starting position.

Count 3. Sit up, turn trunk to left, touch right elbow to left knee.

Count 4. Return to starting position. Score one each time you return to starting position.

6. LEG RAISER (ON EXTENDED ARM)

Starting Position: Body rigidly supported by extended right arm and foot. Left arm is held behind head.

Action: Count 1. Raise left leg high.

Count 2. Return to starting position slowly. Do required number of repetitions. Repeat on other side.

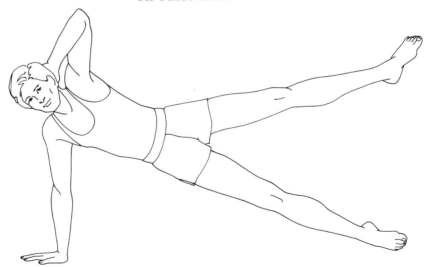

Warm-up exercises	Exercises 1–6 of orientation program	
		Uninterrupted repetitions
Conditioning exercises	1. Toe touch (twist and bend)	30 each side
	2. Sprinter	36
	3. Sitting stretch (alternate)	30
	4. Push-up	50
	5. Sit-up (fingers laced, knees bent)	40
	6. Leg raiser (on extended arm) ..	20 each side
	7. Prone arch (fingers laced)	30
Circulatory activity (choose one each workout)	Jog-run	3 miles
	Rope (skip 2 minutes; rest 30 seconds)	3 series
	Run in place (run 216, hop 30—two cycles)	6 minutes
Water activities	See recommendations in Chapter V.	

Your progress record	1	2	3	4	5	6	7	8	9	10	11	12	13	14	15
Step test (pulse)													Prove-out workouts		

7. PRONE ARCH (FINGERS LACED)

Starting Position: Lie face down, fingers laced behind neck.
Action: Count 1. Arch back, legs, and chest off floor.
Count 2. Extend arms forward.
Count 3. Return hands to behind neck.
Count 4. Flatten body to floor.

Circulatory Activities

Jog-Run   Alternately jog and run the specified distance. Attempt to increase the proportion of time spent running in each succeeding workout.

Rope   Skip or jump rope continuously using any form for 2 minutes and then rest 30 seconds. Repeat 3 times.

Run in Place   Raise each foot at least 4" off floor and jog in place. Count 1 each time left foot touches floor. Complete number of running steps called for in chart, then do specified number of straddle hops. Complete 2 cycles of alternate running and hopping for time specified on the chart.

STRADDLE HOP

Starting Position: At attention.
         Action: Count 1. Swing arms sideward and upward, touching hands above head (arms straight) while simultaneously moving feet sideward and apart in a single jumping motion.
Count 2. Spring back to starting position. Two counts in one hop.

STAYING FIT

After you reach the level of fitness you have decided is best for you, you can keep fit by continuing the workouts for that level.

While it is possible to keep fit with three workouts a week, ideally, exercise should be a daily habit. If you can, by all means continue your workouts on a five-times-a-week basis.

If at any point while reaching for or maintaining your goal, the workouts are interrupted for more than a week, begin again at a lower level. If you have had a serious illness or surgery, check with your physician before you begin again.

BROADENING YOUR PROGRAM

The exercises and activities you have been doing are basic. They are designed only to take you to physical fitness without need for special equipment or facilities.

There are many other activities which, if you wish, you can use to supplement the basic program. You will find them discussed in Chapter V. They include a variety of sports, exercises and activities.

The next chapter discusses supplementary exercise and offers suggestions for taking advantage of many daily opportunities for sound physical activity and maintaining good posture.

Daily Exercises: Anywhere/ Anytime

Now that you have started your physical-fitness program, keep going until you reach the level that is most satisfying and practical for you. Keep this book handy and use it. If your interest lags, read Chapter I again. Rereading about the benefits of physical fitness will spark your enthusiasm once more.

Your progress may seem slow at first, and there will be days when you will not feel like exercising at all, but stick to your schedule. That is the secret of success.

Modern technology constantly tempts us to lead lives of ease, inactivity, and passive participation. This lifestyle is not the way to physical fitness. Regular exercise and activity are as necessary for a healthy body as food and water. Without exercise, the body loses its ability to function properly. You made a tentative commitment to a fuller and more active life by reading this book. But doing the exercises regularly is the way to a full commitment and a healthier body. Follow the suggestions in this book, and you will be well repaid for your efforts.

DAILY OPPORTUNITIES FOR FITNESS

There are many occasions for exercise every day and, by taking advantage of them, you can speed your progress and more easily maintain your top level of fitness. Here are some examples:

Stairs. At least once a day, climb up a flight. As your level of fitness rises, bound up the stairs—two at a time.

Coffee Breaks. Instead of having coffee and a snack, do a few exercises. No need to get into a sweat. Two or three conditioning exercises, that's all. If you lack privacy, do some of the inconspicuous isometric exercises.

Pull-ins. At every opportunity, suck in your abdomen, and hold it taut for a count of five.

Stretch. If you work in a sitting position for long periods, get up occasionally. Stand erect, stretch a bit, and move around.

Rub Away. After a shower or bath, towel yourself vigorously. This is exercise, too, and a great way to stimulate your muscles as well as your skin.

Walk. *Every chance you get!*

WALKING

Walking deserves special emphasis.

Walking is one of the best all-around physical activities. It costs nothing; it is enjoyable; and it benefits more than your muscles. When you walk, your leg muscles "massage" the veins in your legs so that the blood flows more freely back to your heart. The best way to walk is with a brisk step while you breathe deeply and swing your arms.

You probably have more opportunities for a daily walk than you realize. Review your schedule and see where you can allow extra time to catch a train, get to a meeting, or do your shopping on foot.

Whenever you feel tense and nervous, try a walk. The brisker and longer, the better, but even a brief one will relax you. If you have trouble sleeping, a short walk before bed will help cure your insomnia.

Walking is also a wonderful family activity. Once a month or so, why not get the entire family together for a nice, long walk to a local park, scenic area, or even through your own town?

But the important thing is to walk at every opportunity!

ISOMETRICS

Isometric contraction exercises are great anywhere and anytime because they take only a few seconds and require no special equipment. They are an easy way to strengthen muscles.

The idea of isometrics is to work out a muscle by pushing or pulling against an immovable object, such as a wall, or by pitting it against the opposition of another muscle. The muscles are worked harder than they normally are and become stronger. Research does indicate that one hard six- to eight-second isometric contraction per workout can, over a period of six months, produce stronger muscles.

The exercises illustrated and described in the following pages cover the major large muscle groups of the body.

You can do isometrics in the order shown on the following pages, or you can skip around as you please. And you do not have to do them all in one isometric session. A few at a time is fine. One or two in the morning, others at various times during the day— whenever you have half a minute or even less to spare.

For each contraction, maintain the tension for *no more than eight seconds*. Do little breathing during a contraction; breathe deeply between contractions. And start easily. Do *not* apply the maximum effort in the beginning. For the first three or four weeks, you should exert only about one-half of what you think is your maximum force. Use the first three or four seconds to build up to this degree of force and the remaining four or five seconds to hold it. After the first three or four weeks, you can gradually increase the force until you reach the maximum. It takes about six weeks to build up to the maximum force.

If you feel pain, that means you are applying too much force; reduce the amount immediately. If the pain continues, stop isometrics for a week or two. Try again, but with about fifty percent of the maximum effort. If the pain does not recur, you can go on gradually building toward the maximum effort.

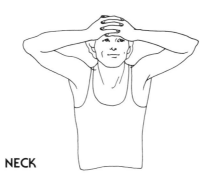

NECK

Starting Position: Sit or stand. Interlace fingers and place hands on forehead.

Action: Exert a strong forward push with head. Use hands to resist.

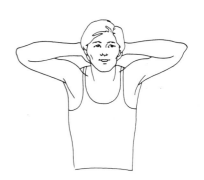

Starting Position: Sit or stand, with interlaced fingers of hands behind head.

Action: Push head backward while exerting a forward pull with hands.

Starting Position: Sit or stand, with palm of left hand on left side of head.

Action: Push with left hand while resisting with head and neck. Reverse using right hand on right side of head.

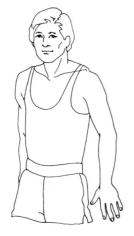

UPPER BODY

Starting Position: Stand, back to wall, hands at sides, palms toward wall.

Action: Press hands backward against wall, keeping arms straight.

Starting Position: Stand, facing wall, hands at sides, palms toward wall.

Action: Press hands forward against wall, keeping arms straight.

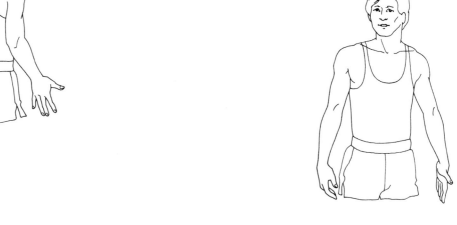

Starting Position: Stand in doorway or with side against wall, arms at sides, palms toward legs.

Action: Press hand(s) outward against wall or doorframe, keeping arms straight.

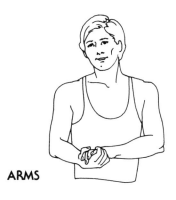

ARMS

Starting Position: Stand with feet slightly apart. Flex right elbow, close to body, palm up. Place left hand over right.

Action: Forcibly attempt to curl right arm upward, while giving equally strong resistance with the left hand. Repeat with left arm.

ARMS AND CHEST

Starting Position: Stand with feet comfortably spaced, knees slightly bent. Clasp hands, palms together, close to chest.

Action: Press hands together and hold.

Starting Position: Stand with feet slightly apart, knees slightly bent. Grip fingers, arms close to chest.

Action: Pull against finger grip.

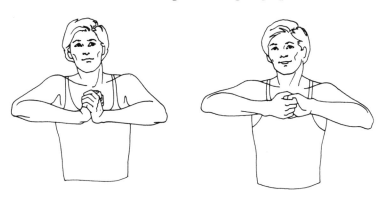

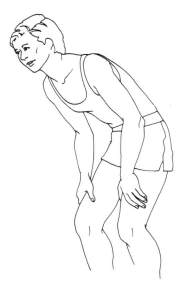

ABDOMINAL

Starting Position: Stand, knees slightly flexed, hands resting on knees.

Action: Contract abdominal muscles.

LOWER BACK, BUTTOCKS AND BACKS OF THIGHS

Starting Position: Lie face down, arms at sides, palms up, legs placed under bed or other heavy object.

Action: With both hips flat on floor, raise one leg, keeping knee straight so that heel pushes hard against the resistance above. Repeat with opposite leg.

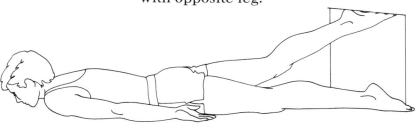

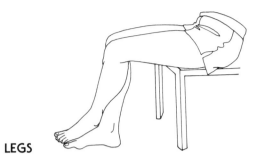

LEGS

Starting Position: Sit in chair with left ankle crossed over right, feet resting on floor, legs bent at 90 degree angle.

Action: Forcibly attempt to straighten right leg while resisting with the left. Repeat with opposite leg.

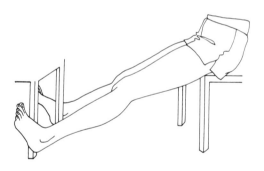

INNER AND OUTER THIGHS

Starting Position: Sit, legs extended with each ankle pressed against the outside of sturdy chair legs.

Action: Keep legs straight and pull toward one another firmly. For outer thigh muscles, place ankles inside chair legs and exert pressure outward.

WATER ACTIVITIES

Swimming is a valuable activity for almost everyone. When the body is submerged in water, blood circulation increases automatically. When there is water pressure against the body, the lungs ventilate better. With well-planned activity, both circulation and ventilation increase still more.

The water exercises described on the following page can be used either as supplements to, or as replacements for, the circulatory activities of the basic program. The goals for each of the five levels are shown in the chart below.

WOMEN

Level	1	2	3	4	5
Bobs	10	15	20	50	100
Swim	5 min.	10 min.	15 min.		
Interval swimming				25 yds. (Repeat 10 times.)	25 yds. (Repeat 20 times.)

MEN

Level	1	2	3	4	5
Bobs	10	15	25	75	125
Swim	5 min.	10 min.	15 min.		
Interval swimming				25 yds. (Repeat 20 times.)	50 yds. (Repeat 20 times.)

Bobbing

Starting Position: Face out of water.

Action: Count 1. Take a breath. Count 2. Submerge while exhaling until feet touch bottom. Count 3. Push up from bottom to surface while continuing to exhale. Three counts to one bob.

Swimming

Use any type of stroke. Swim continuously for the time specified.

Interval Swimming

Use any type of stroke. Swim at a moderate speed for the specified distance. Either swim slowly back to your starting point or climb out of the pool and walk back. Repeat this the number of times specified.

WEIGHT TRAINING

Weight training also is an excellent method of developing muscular strength—and muscular endurance. Where equipment is available, it may be used as a supplement to the conditioning exercises.

Because of the great variety of weight training exercises, there will be no attempt to describe them here. Both barbells and weighted dumbbells—complete with instructions—are available at most sporting goods stores. A good rule to follow in deciding the maximum weight you should lift is to select a weight you can lift six times without strain.

SPORTS

Soccer, basketball, handball, squash, ice hockey and other sports that require sustained effort can be valuable aids to building circulatory endurance.

But if you have been sedentary, it's important to pace yourself carefully in such sports, and it may even be advisable to avoid them until you are well along in your physical conditioning program. That does not mean you should avoid all sports.

There are many excellent conditioning and circulatory activities in which the amount of exertion is easily controlled and in which you can progress at your own rate. Bicycling is one example. Others include hiking, skating, tennis, running, cross-country skiing, rowing, canoeing, water skiing and skindiving.

You can take part in these sports at any point in the program, if you begin slowly. But do not play so vigorously that you become over-tired.

On days when you get a good workout in sports you can skip part or all of your exercise program. Use your own judgment.

If you have engaged in a sport that exercises the legs and stimulates the heart and lungs—such as skating—you could skip the circulatory activity for that day, but you still should do some of the conditioning and stretching exercises for the upper body. On the other hand, weight lifting is an excellent conditioning activity, but it should be supplemented with running or one of the other circulatory exercises.

Whatever your favorite sport, you will find your enjoyment increased by improved fitness. Every weekend athlete should invest in frequent workouts.

POSTURE

There is a relationship between good posture and physical fitness. One helps the other.

When your posture is good, you are less likely to cramp your internal organs. Blood also circulates more freely, and your muscles do not tense up as quickly. Physical conditioning strengthens your muscles. Strong muscles allow you to correct poor posture habits. Good posture allows you to keep your muscles strong.

For good posture, the gravity centers of your feet, legs, hips, trunk, shoulders, and head must be in a vertical line. When you are standing, a side view should show an invisible straight line running from your earlobe through the tip of your shoulder, down to the middle of your hips, just back of the kneecap, and ending in front of the outer ankle bone.

STANDING

1. Feet parallel, about 6" apart.
2. Head high, as if balancing a book.
3. Chest out.
4. Stomach and hips firm.
5. Abdomen and back as flat as possible.

6. Knees very lightly flexed, not stiffly locked.
7. Weight evenly distributed on both feet, most of it on balls of feet.

SITTING

1. Sit tall and back, with hips touching the back of the chair, feet flat on floor.
2. Chest out, back of neck nearly in line with upper back.
3. When writing, lean forward from the hips so you keep head and shoulders in line.

The position of your hips is a good way to check your posture. They should rest squarely on your legs. There should be no forward or backward tilt. Flabby abdominal muscles and excess weight, particularly in the abdominal region, can cause poor posture. Weak abdominal muscles let the internal organs drop so that the abdomen protrudes. This is the cause of the stomach "paunch" so many overweight people have. The paunch upsets their center of gravity. As the paunch pulls them forward, they compensate by leaning back and bending their knees slightly. Their spines curve inward, and they carry themselves with an "old man's stance."

Wearing very high heels too often can produce the same effect in women, even young women. High-heeled shoes make the muscles in the calves and the thighs short. When these muscles are short, wearing low-heeled shoes or going barefoot is uncomfortable.

Forward head, or "poked neck," is another common result of poor posture. When the head is out of line, some other part of the body compensates and also moves out of line.

Good posture is not difficult. All it takes is practice. Give your body a treat; carry it properly. In return, you will find that you not only look better, but that you also feel better.

WALKING

1. Knees and ankles limber, toes pointed straight ahead.
2. Head and chest high.
3. Swing legs directly forward from hip joints.
4. Push feet off the ground—don't shuffle.
5. Swing shoulders and arms freely and easily.

Exercises for
Senior Citizens

THE ACTIVE LIFE

The years in late life, particularly those of the post-retirement period, should be happy years. But the full promise of this stage of life comes only to those who are healthy, alert, and active. The later years can be truly rewarding if you have the energy and zest to use them well.

The way to *keep* lively is to *be* lively; the way to stay active is to move. Energy makes energy, and the only way to develop the capacity to expend more and more energy is to keep increasingly active.

It is nice to come into retirement with a bankroll of physical resources, just as it is comforting to have sufficient income. Some folks hit their sixties with plenty of bounce, having kept fit and active throughout their adult years. And this is like having great wealth.

Even if you have let too many years slip by when good intentions of keeping fit were sacrificed to other demands of life, fortunately you can still pick up at some level of physical performance and work yourself up several notches. The programs described here are to help bring you from your present level of fitness up to a higher one. Just how fit you would like to be is your choice, but why not aim to be as fit as you are physically able to be?

But why strive for more "bounce to the ounce" in your retirement years? Because you will be able to keep your health, and when you are sick, you will be able to recover faster.

There is another reason why fitness is important. Physically active and able people usually have a positive feeling about themselves. They also possess a degree of physical courage that propels them into interesting and stimulating experiences. They move with grace and ease; they generally present a trim, attractive, and self-confident figure.

Perhaps the greatest benefit of maintaining physical fitness is the degree of independence it affords. This is a quality to be most prized in the later years. There is a great psychological and financial advantage in having the ability to plan and do things without depending upon relatives, friends, or hired help. To drive your own car, to succeed with do-it-yourself projects rather than trying to find and pay someone else for the service, to go and come as you please, to be an aid rather than a liability in emergencies—these are forms of personal freedom well worth working for.

HOW EXERCISE PROMOTES DYNAMIC FITNESS

Efficiency and Endurance of the Heart and Lungs

Keeping your heart, lungs, and blood vessels working properly is one of the most important aspects of fitness in your retirement years.

More and more evidence from scientific research points to the importance of regular physical activity in maintaining good circulation and respiration. To stay healthy, you have to keep moving.

Muscular Strength and Endurance

Muscles grow in size and strength only if they are used. If they are not, the muscles become soft, flabby, and weak. While strength does decrease with advancing years, the rate of decline can be lessened by keeping the muscles toned through regular exercise. With a program such as this one, you can gradually improve your muscular strength.

Balance

It is important that your balance mechanism be kept in the best possible state. A poor sense of balance is a hazard for anyone but especially for older people. A fall can result in broken bones and a long recovery period. Regular physical activity can help keep the balance mechanism up to par.

Flexibility

Few of us give any thought to our body joints until a touch of arthritis develops. Yet arthritis can be delayed, or even avoided, if the joints are exercised regularly. This program is designed to help keep your joints flexible.

And, too, just because you are not as young as you used to be is no reason to stop bending, stretching, and reaching. You may think you are doing your body a favor when you keep shelves low and appliances within easy reach, but you are not. Flex your joints as often as possible.

Coordination and Agility

A well-coordinated individual should be able to move gracefully; to change direction quickly and safely. Vision and motion should work together. A high level of coordination and agility is still necessary as you grow older, especially if you drive. It is necessary, too, if you are to enjoy the recreation you plan for yourself.

PRINCIPLES OF EXERCISE AND FITNESS PROGRAMMING

Physical fitness can be improved by gradually increasing the amount of time spent exercising, but it is necessary to move in easy stages. The enthusiast who tackles a keep-fit program too fast and too strenuously soon gives up. Speed is not important; what is important is that you stick to your program. Physical activity has got to be maintained to achieve the full benefits, but exercise has a cumulative effect. Every little bit counts.

For example, every movement uses calories, so the way to burn up calories is to move. Even though certain actions, such as a short walk, may not use many calories at the time, a number of short walks in the course of a day can use up a fair-sized total. Similarly, the organs, joints, and muscles benefit from every move you make. Therefore, try to step up activity throughout your day while you follow your exercise program.

At all ages, but particularly in later years, it is important to prepare your body for vigorous activity by "warming up." Anyone, and especially older people, should avoid sudden strenuous activity. A warm-up period is essential. Running in place is a good way to warm up. Start slowly and gradually increase your speed until your pulse rate, breathing, and body temperature are higher. It is also a good idea to do some easy stretching, pulling, and rotating exercises during the warm-up period.

Periods of vigorous exercise should be followed with periods of less strenuous exercise. "Put the pressure on" for a while and then release it. By gradually increasing the stressful interval and reducing the less vigorous interval, you improve your physical condition. This principle of "interval training" can be applied to many forms of exercise and is particularly adaptable to walking, jogging, and swimming.

The proper way to advance in strength and physical condition is to put increasing workloads on your system. This is called the "overload principle." Challenge yourself little by little toward improved performance by increasing the amount of exercise performed or the speed at which you perform it. For example, if you repeat an exercise five times, a certain amount of work has been done and value derived. The next step is to perform the exercise six times, and then gradually increase the number until you can do it, say, ten times with ease.

Unless the overload principle is used, only a minimum amount of good is achieved. This is why it is important to follow a gradual, progressive plan.

Exercise is, of course, only one part of being active and physically fit. Regular medical and dental care, a good diet, and rest are all important to a "balanced life." Take them all into consideration.

Now—to your fitness program!

YOUR EXERCISE PROGRAM—LEVEL ONE, LEVEL TWO, OR LEVEL THREE?

This program has three levels graded according to their difficulty or the amount of stress involved. They are identified as Level One, Level Two, and Level Three. Level One is the easiest, Level Two is more advanced, and Level Three is the most difficult and sustained. They let you start where you should, and they provide for an easy progression as you improve your physical condition.

Each of these three exercise programs is designed to give you a balanced workout, as you will use all major muscle groups. Doing your program regularly will lead to improvement in the various areas of physical fitness, especially in functioning of the heart and lungs.

As you become better at the exercises in your program, you should increase the number of repetitions of certain exercises, and increase the duration and speed of walking and jogging.

As you increase the number of repetitions and handle more complicated and demanding exercises, you can move up to the next level with new confidence and a growing feeling of well-being.

How do you know where to start? Are you Level One, Level Two, or Level Three?

First, you should ask your physician for advice. Discuss your plans with your own doctor (or public health clinic physician) and follow his recommendations. Take this book along to show him. Ask him to review the program recommended here and to advise you accordingly. Also give yourself the following simple tests to determine your present condition and your exercise tolerance. In other words, find out just what kind of shape you are in.

The tests will help you select your appropriate exercise level and pace. Keep in mind that there are wide variations in physical performance. Your own individual physical condition must dictate your personal exercise program.

Check yourself in easy stages. First, try the walk test below.

WALK TEST

The idea behind this walk test is to determine how long, up to ten minutes, you can walk briskly, without undue difficulty or discomfort, on a level surface. It is preferable to take the test outdoors, but walking around the room indoors will do if necessary.

If you can finish three minutes, but no more, you should begin your daily exercise program with Level One.

If you can go beyond three minutes, but not quite to ten minutes, you can warm up at Level One for a week or two, and then move up to Level Two.

If you can breeze through the whole ten minutes, you are ready for bigger things. Rest awhile, or wait until the next day, and then take Walk-Jog Test #1.

A note of caution: If you develop nausea, trembling, extreme breathlessness, pounding headache, or chest pains while taking these tests, stop immediately. These symptoms indicate that you have gone beyond your present level of exercise tolerance. If the symptoms do not pass within five minutes, discontinue the program and check with your physician.

WALK-JOG TEST #1

This test consists of alternately walking fifty steps and jogging fifty steps for a total of six minutes. Read instructions under Exercise #2 on page 126 and the section on jogging (page 185) before starting this test.

Walk at the rate of 120 steps per minute; that is, your left foot strikes the ground once each second. *Jog* at the rate of 144 steps per minute; your left foot hits the ground eighteen times every fifteen seconds. Time your walking and jogging intervals for fifteen seconds occasionally to check your pace.

If you stop this test before the six minutes are up, plan your schedule of exercises at Level Two.

If you complete the six-minute walk-jog test without difficulty, you can probably undertake Level Three. It might be well, however, to *warm up* for a week or two on Level Two.

If you can do this test without difficulty and feel you are capable of a more rigorous trial, wait twenty-four hours and then take Walk-Jog Test #2.

WALK-JOG TEST #2

This test consists of alternately walking 100 steps and jogging 100 steps for a total of ten minutes. Follow the directions and use the same rates of speed—walking and jogging—as described for Walk-Jog Test #1.

If you complete this ten-minute test without difficulty, you can obviously handle Level Three.

KEEP AN EXERCISE SCHEDULE

Now that you've tested yourself and determined where to begin, set aside thirty minutes to an hour a day for a planned program of physical activity. You should consider your exercises just as important as proper food and rest.

The exercises in this program are not graded separately for men and women but are tailored to individuals. A couple can do the exercises together. More than likely, however, a man who has been active can start at a higher level or progress faster than most of the women who undertake the program.

Begin *very easily* and increase the tempo and number of repetitions *very gradually*. This will keep stiffness and soreness to a minimum. If you do get a little stiff during the first few days, don't let it slow you down; the stiffness will soon be overcome and it is an indication that you *needed* the activity.

Follow the directions for your exercise exactly. If, for example, you are at Level One and a particular exercise should be performed only twice as a starter, stop after two repetitions—even though you may feel you can do many more. A warm-up is built into each exercise series. Therefore, the exercises should be performed in the order presented to give best results.

Keep a record of the exercises you do, and how many times you repeat them. The little extra time required to keep a record of your activities and to set more and more challenging goals for yourself is well spent. A fitness program should be carefully designed and carefully followed. The best way to keep track of each day's performance is to write it down. The exercise schedules outlined in this book will be more beneficial to you if you keep good records.

One way of adding to the fun of your exercise program is to play music while you are exercising. You can select lively tunes and find music that fits the tempo of the various movements. This is particularly interesting when walking or jogging indoors. Some people also enjoy exercising while watching TV.

You can exercise with family and friends. Many groups get together in each other's homes or at a local center or club.

Wear comfortable clothing. Avoid tight-fitting, restrictive clothes, although, if you feel more comfortable wearing foundation garments, do so. Shorts or slacks, T-shirts or short-sleeved blouses are usually desirable. Wear well-fitting shoes with nonslip soles and low (or no) heels.

SPECIFIC INSTRUCTIONS FOR INDIVIDUAL PROGRAMS—LEVEL ONE, LEVEL TWO, AND LEVEL THREE

Level One

Try to complete the entire sequence without undue rest periods between exercises, but of course, rest awhile if you feel overtaxed. One indication of your improved condition is the ability to go through the workout in less and less time (up to a point), which means doing the exercises at a faster pace and resting for shorter periods between exercises. Never let the effort to increase speed cause jerky movements or otherwise interfere with correct performance of the exercise.

For the first week at least do only the suggested minimum. If you find that even this is strenuous or if you feel tired at the end of the week, continue at the same pace for another week.

After the first week, or as you are ready, in each exercise where a range of repetitions is shown, increase the minimum by *one*. Do this number, but no more, the second week. (If you need to stay at the lowest count, as explained above, do not increase the count at all.) In the following weeks, gradually increase the number of repetitions as you feel you can. Most people should take three to four weeks to reach the highest counts in the Level One program.

After you reach the point where you can do the highest number of repetitions shown for each exercise, continue on Level One until you can complete the whole series without resting between exercises.

When you can do this for three days in a row, move on to Level Two.

Level Two

When you are ready for Level Two, proceed as you did for Level One. That is, start by doing each exercise the minimum number of times suggested.

Most people should remain at Level Two for three to five weeks before moving to Level Three.

After you pass your "prove-out" test by

performing all of the Level Two exercises at the highest frequency shown without resting in between for three consecutive workouts, move on to Level Three.

Level Three

Follow the same directions as for the Level One and Level Two programs. Start slowly; step up activity gradually.

When you reach the upper limits of the Level Three exercises and can go through the workout without stopping on three straight days, you are ready to tackle bigger things. Continue with the exercises in this book, gradually increasing the number and speed of repetitions, the distances walked and jogged, and also engage in more sports and recreational activities; or turn to the fitness programs for men and women (Chapters III and IV), which include more difficult exercises, and advance to Level One without going through the orientation level.

IMPORTANT NOTE Most, but *not all,* of the exercises illustrated on the following pages are included in all three exercise programs—Level One, Level Two, and Level Three—but the same order is *not* followed in the three programs.

Do only those exercises included in your program level.

Perform your exercises in the order indicated for your program.

ORDER OF EXERCISES

Level One	Level Two	Level Three

Illustrations of each exercise and figures for number of repetitions or length of time to perform it appear on pages 132–148. Where two figures are given, start at the lower figure; gradually increase the repetitions or duration over a period of days or weeks until you can perform the higher number.

Level One	Level Two	Level Three
Walk 2 minutes	Walk 3 minutes	Alternate Walk (50 steps) Jog (50) 3 minutes
Bend and Stretch	Bend and Stretch	
Rotate Head	Rotate Head	Bend and Stretch
Body Bender	Body Bender	Rotate Head
Wall Press	Wall Press	Body Bender
Arm Circles	Arm Circles	Wall Press
Wing Stretcher	Half Knee Bend	Arm Circles
Walk 2–5 minutes	Wing Stretcher	Half Knee Bend
Lying Leg Bend	Wall Push-Away	Wing Stretcher
Angel Stretch	Walk 5 minutes	Alternate Walk (50 steps) Jog (50) 3 minutes
Walk a Straight Line	Lying Leg Bend	
Wall Push-Away	Angel Stretch	Leg Raise and Bend
Side Leg Raise	Walk the Beam (2-inch by 6-inch beam)	Angel Stretch
Head and Shoulder Curl		Walk the Beam (2-inch by 4-inch beam)
Alternate Walk (50 steps) Jog (10) 1–3 minutes	Knee Pushup	Hop
	Side Leg Raise	Knee Push Up
Walk 1–3 minutes	Head and Shoulder Curl (arms crossed on chest)	Side Leg Raise
	Diver's Stance	Head and Shoulder Curl (hands clasped behind neck)
	Alternate Walk (50 steps) Jog (25) 3–6 minutes	Stork Stand
	Walk 1–3 minutes	Alternate Walk (50 steps) Jog (50) 5 minutes, gradually increasing to walk 100 steps—jog 100
		Walk 3 minutes

EXERCISES

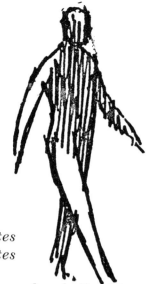

1. WALK

Level 1: 2 minutes
Level 2: 3 minutes

Starting Position: Stand erect, balanced on balls of feet.
Action: Begin walking briskly on a level space, preferably outdoors, but walking around the room will do if necessary.
Value: A good warm-up exercise, loosening muscles, and preparing you for your full exercise schedule.

Arms flexed

2. ALTERNATE WALK-JOG

Flatfooted

Level 3 only at this time
Alternately walk 50 steps and jog 50—for about 3 minutes

Starting Position: Same as for walking but with arms held flexed, forearms generally parallel to the ground.
Action: Jogging is a form of slow running. Begin walking for 50 steps, then shift to a slow run

with easy strides, landing lightly each time on the heel of the foot and transfer weight to the whole foot in flatfooted style. (This is heel-toe running, in contrast to the sprint, in which the runner stays on balls of his feet.) Arms should move loosely and freely from the shoulders in opposition to legs. Breathing should be deep but not labored to point of gasping.

Value: Good warm-up for more advanced exercises. Good for legs and circulation.

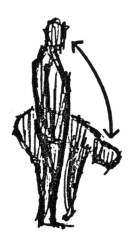

3. BEND AND STRETCH

Level 1: Repeat 2 to 10 times
Level 2: Repeat 10 times
Level 3: Repeat 10 times

Starting Position: Stand erect, feet shoulder width apart.

Action: Count 1. Bend trunk forward and down, flexing knees. Stretch gently in attempt to touch fingers to toes or floor.
Count 2. Return to starting position.
Note: Do slowly, stretch and relax at intervals rather than in rhythm.

Value: Helps loosen and stretch most muscles of body; helps relaxation; aids in warm-up for more vigorous exercise.

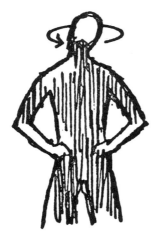

4. ROTATE HEAD

Level 1: Repeat 2 to 10 times each way
Level 2: Repeat 10 times each way
Level 3: Repeat 10 times each way

Starting Position: Stand erect, feet shoulder width apart, hands on hips.

Action: Count 1. Slowly rotate the head in a full circle from left to right.

Count 2. Slowly rotate head in the opposite direction.

Note: Use slow, smooth motion; close eyes to help avoid losing balance or getting dizzy.

Value: Helps loosen and relax muscles of the neck, and firm up throat and chin line.

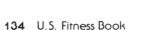

5. BODY BENDER

Level 1: Repeat 2 to 5 times
Level 2: Repeat 5 to 10 times
Level 3: Repeat 10 times

Starting Position: Stand with feet shoulder width apart, hands extended overhead, fingertips touching.
Action: Count 1. Bend trunk slowly sideward to left as far as possible, keeping hands together and arms straight (do not bend elbows).
Count 2. Return to starting position.
Counts 3 and 4. Repeat to the right.
Value: Stretches arm, trunk, and leg muscles.

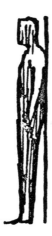

6. WALL PRESS

Level 1: Repeat 2 to 5 times
Level 2: Repeat 5 times
Level 3: Repeat 5 times

Starting Position: Stand erect, head not bent forward or backward, back against wall, heels about 3 inches away from wall.
Action: Count 1. Pull in the abdominal muscles and press the small of the back tight against the wall. Hold for six seconds.
Count 2. Relax and return to starting position.
Note: Keep entire back in contact with wall on Count 1 and do not tilt the head backward.
Value: Promotes good body alignment and posture. Strengthens abdominal muscles.

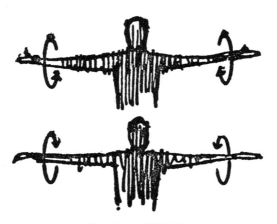

7. ARM CIRCLES

Level 1: Repeat 5 each way
Level 2: Repeat 5 to 10 each way
Level 3: Repeat 10 to 15 each way

Starting Position: Stand erect, arms extended sideward at shoulder height, palms up.
Action: Rotate hands clockwise. Keep head erect. Turn palms down and rotate hands counterclockwise.
Value: Helps to keep the shoulder joints flexible; strengthens muscles of shoulders.

8. HALF KNEE BEND

Level 1: Skip this exercise at this time
Level 2: Repeat 5 to 10 times
Level 3: Repeat 10 to 15 times

Starting Position: Stand erect, hands on hips.
Action: Count 1. Bend knees halfway while extend-

ing arms forward, palms down. Keep heels on floor.

Count 2. Return to starting position.

Value: Firms up leg muscles and stretches muscles in front of legs. Helps improve balance.

9. WING STRETCHER

Level 1: Repeat 2 to 5 times
Level 2: Repeat 5 to 10 times
Level 3: Repeat 10 to 20 times

Starting Position: Stand erect, bend arms in front of chest, extended fingertips touching and elbows at shoulder height.

Counts 1, 2, 3. Pull elbows back as far as possible, keeping arms at shoulder height and returning to starting position each time.

Count 4. Swing arms outward and sideward, shoulder height, palms up, and return to starting position.

Note: This is a bouncy, rhythmic action, counting "one-and-two-and-three-and-four."

Value: Strengthens muscles of upper back and shoulders; stretches chest muscles. .Helps promote good posture and prevent "dowager hump."

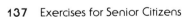

NOTE: At this point in sequence:
   Level 1 now return to Walk (Exercise #1) and walk two to five minutes.
   Level 2 return to Walk (Exercise #1) and walk five minutes.
   Level 3 return to Alternate Walk-Jog (Exercise #2) and walk fifty steps, jog fifty for three minutes.

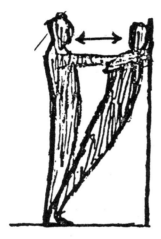

10. WALL PUSH-AWAY

Level 2 only, at this time
Repeat exercise 10 times
Then walk for 5 minutes

Starting Position: Stand erect, feet about six inches apart, facing a wall and arms straight in front, palms on wall, bearing weight slightly.

Action: Count 1. Bend elbows and lower body slowly toward wall, meanwhile turning head to the side, until cheek almost touches the wall.

Count 2. Push against wall with the arms and return to the starting position.

Note: Keep heels on floor throughout the exercise.

Value: Increases strength of arm, shoulder, and upper-back muscles. Stretches muscles in chest and back of legs.

11. LYING LEG BEND

Level 1: Repeat 2 to 5 times, each leg
Level 2: Repeat 5 to 10 times, each leg
Level 3: Skip this exercise

Starting Position: Lie on back, legs extended, feet together, arms at sides.

Action: Count 1. Bend left knee and move left foot toward buttocks, keeping foot in light contact with floor.

Count 2. Move knee toward chest as far as possible, using abdominal, hip, and leg muscles; *then* clasp knee with both hands and pull slowly toward chest.

Count 3. Return to position at end of count 1.

Count 4. Return to starting position.

Note: After completing desired number of repetitions with left leg, repeat the exercise using right leg.

Value: Improves flexibility of knee and hip joints; and strengthens abdominal and hip muscles.

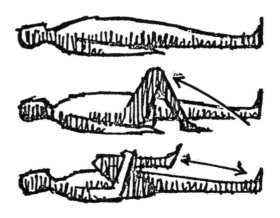

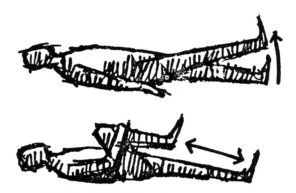

12. LEG RAISE AND BEND

Level 3: Repeat 2 to 5 times   Level 3 only
After completing desired number with left
leg, do exercise with right leg

Starting Position: Lie on back, legs extended, feet together, arms at sides.

Action: Count 1. Raise extended left leg about 12 inches off the floor.

Count 2. Bend knee and move knee toward chest as far as possible, using abdominal, hip, and leg muscles; *then* clasp knee with both hands and pull slowly toward chest.

Count 3. Return to position at end of count 1.

Count 4. Return to starting position.

Value: Improves flexibility of knee and hip joints; strengthens abdominal muscles.

13. ANGEL STRETCH

Level 1: Repeat 2 to 5 times
Level 2: Repeat 5 times
Level 3: Repeat 5 times

Starting Position: Lie on back, legs straight, feet together; arms extended at sides.

Action: Count 1. Move arms and legs outward along the floor to a "spread-eagle" position. Slide —do not raise—arms and legs.

Count 2. Return to starting position.

Note: Throughout the exercise try to compress the lower back against the floor by tightening the abdominal muscles. Do not arch the lower back.

Value: Stretches muscles of arms, legs, trunk, aids posture; improves strength of abdominal muscles.

14. WALK A STRAIGHT LINE

Level 1: Walk for 10 feet
Level 2 and Level 3: Skip this, do Walk the Beam (#15) instead

Starting Position: Stand erect with left foot along a straight line. Arms held away from body to aid balance.

Action: Count 1. Walk the length of the straight line by putting the right foot in front of the left foot with right heel touching left toe, and then placing the feet alternately one in front of the other, heel-to-toe.

Count 2. Return to the starting point by walking backward along the line, alternately placing one foot behind the other, toe-to-heel.

Value: Improves balance; helps posture.

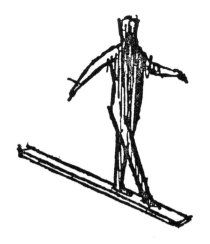

15. WALK THE BEAM

Level 2: Walk 10 feet on 2" x 6" board
Level 3: Walk 10 feet on 2" x 4" board

Starting Position: Stand erect with left foot on board, long axis of foot in line with board.

Action: Count 1. Walk the length of the board by putting the right foot in front of the left foot with right heel touching left toe, and then placing the feet alternately one in front of the other, heel-to-toe.

Count 2. Return to the starting point by walking backward along the length of the board, alternately placing one foot behind the other, toe-to-heel.

Note: The board is placed flat on the floor, not on the 2" edge.

Value: Improves balance; helps posture.

NOTE: At this point in sequence:

Level 1 perform Half Knee Bend (#8) repeating it two to five times; Wall Push-Away

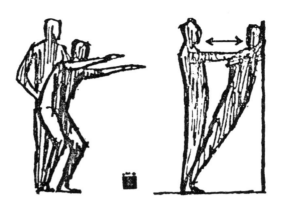

(#10) repeating two to ten times; then skip #15, 16, and 17, moving to #18 next.

16. HOP

Level 3: Hop 5 times on each foot
Level 3 only

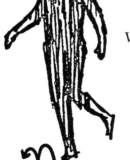

Starting Position: Stand erect, weight on right foot, left leg bent slightly at the knee, and left foot held a few inches off the floor; arms held sideward slightly away from the body to aid balance.

Action: Count 1. Hop on right foot, moving a few inches forward each hop.

Note: Do the desired number of hops on right leg, then change to left leg and hop.

Value: Improves balance, strengthens extensor muscles of leg and foot; increases circulation.

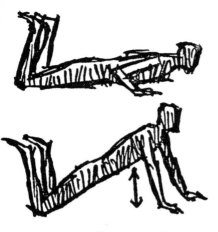

17. KNEE PUSHUP

Level 2: Repeat 1 to 3 times
Level 3: Repeat 3 to 6 times

Starting Position: Lie on floor, face down, legs together, knees bent with feet raised off floor, hands on floor under shoulders, palms down.

Action: Count 1. Push upper body off floor until arms are fully extended and body is in straight line from head to knees.
Count 2. Return to starting position.

Value: Strengthens muscles of arms, shoulders, and trunk.

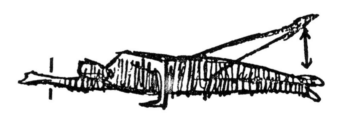

18. SIDE LEG RAISE

Level 1: Repeat 2 to 5 times each leg
Level 2: Repeat 5 to 10 times
Level 3: Repeat 10 times

Starting Position: Right side of body on floor, head resting on right arm.

Count 1. Lift left leg sideward about 30 inches off floor.

Count 2. Return to starting position.

Note: Using the left leg, repeat this exercise the desired number of times.

Value: Helps improve flexibility of the hip joint and strengthens lateral muscles of trunk and hip.

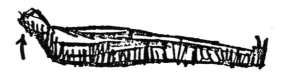

19. HEAD AND SHOULDER CURL

Level 1: Repeat 2 to 5 times; hold each for 4 seconds

Starting Position: Lie on back, legs straight, feet together, arms extended along the front of the legs with palms resting lightly on the thighs.

Action: Count 1. Tighten abdominal muscles and lift head and shoulders so that shoulders are about 10 inches off the floor. Meanwhile slide arms along the legs, keeping them extended. Then hold the position for 4 seconds.

Count 2. Return slowly to starting position, keeping abdominal muscles tight until shoulders and head rest on floor. Relax.

Note: Level 1: Skip exercises #20 and #21.

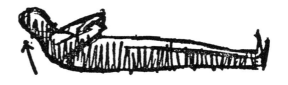

19. HEAD AND SHOULDER CURL

Level 2: Repeat 5 times; hold each for 6 seconds

Same as Level 1 except on starting position arms are crossed over chest (kept in that position throughout).

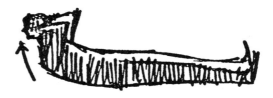

19. HEAD AND SHOULDER CURL

Level 3: Repeat 5 times; hold each for 10 seconds

Same as Level 1, except on starting position, hands are clasped behind the neck (held that way throughout).
Note: The head should lead in a "curling" motion, chin tucked to chest, back rounded, not arched.

Value: Excellent for improving abdominal strength and stretching back muscles.

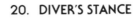

20. DIVER'S STANCE

Level 2 only—hold position for 10 seconds

Starting Position: Stand erect, feet slightly apart, arms at sides.
Action: Rise on toes and bring arms upward and forward so that they extend parallel with the floor, palms down. When this position is attained, close eyes and hold balance for 10 seconds.
Note: Head should be straight and body should be held firmly throughout.
Value: Improves balance; strengthens extensor muscles of feet and legs; helps maintain good posture.

21. STORK STAND

Level 3 only—hold position 10 seconds on each leg

Starting Position: Stand erect, feet slightly apart, hands on hips, head straight.
Action: Transfer weight to the left foot and bend right knee, bringing the sole of the right foot to the inner side of the left knee. When this position is reached, close eyes and hold for 10 seconds.
Note: After holding on left leg, change to the right leg and repeat.
Value: Improves balance.

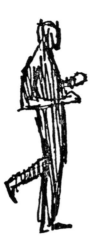

22. ALTERNATE WALK-JOG

(This is a repetition of exercise #2.)
Level 1: Walk 50 steps, jog 10. 1 to 3 minutes
Level 2: Walk 50 steps, jog 25. 3 to 6 minutes
Level 3: Begin walk 50 steps, jog 50. Gradually increase to walk 100 steps, jog 100. Continue for 5 minutes

Value: Provides an interval of exercise for circulatory system, and for strengthening leg muscles.

23. WALK

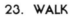

This is a repetition of exercise #1; it ends your daily workout
Level 1: Walk 1 to 3 minutes
Level 2: Walk 1 to 3 minutes
Level 3: Walk 3 minutes

Value: Tapering off, as heart rate, breathing, body heat, and other functions return to normal.

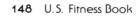

ALTERNATIVES TO YOUR DAILY EXERCISE SCHEDULE

If you can enroll in a keep-fit program at the Y, at a school, or the local recreation center, you can skip your home-exercise routine on those meeting days.

If you can take part in a sport, by all means do so. Swimming is an excellent activity if you really swim. Take advantage of any opportunities you may have to swim regularly. Hiking, bicycling, tennis, or similar sports are also valuable.

On days when you participate in sports, you can substitute the sport for your home-exercise routine, or better still, add it to your day's activity. But make sure, if you substitute it, that the exercise involved in the sport equals your regular workout. Incidentally, by doing your home exercises, you can keep in shape for an occasional opportunity to participate in a sport, and also avoid soreness, stiffness, injury, or overfatigue.

Other forms of active recreation should be worked into your daily life whenever possible. Such activities as gardening, fishing, archery, horseshoes, Ping-Pong, shuffleboard, a family outing, an evening of social or square dancing are not only fun, but will also help you keep vigorous. Age need not be a barrier to participation. These activities should be added to, not substituted for, your daily exercise.

STEPPED-UP DAILY ACTIVITIES

To the daily exercise schedule and your supplementary recreation add a little more action. Gradually, day by day, find ways to move *more* rather than *less*. Walk to the neighborhood store instead of driving (or being driven). Walk down a flight of stairs instead of taking the elevator: When you are back in shape, walk *up* the stairs.

In today's sedentary world, you need to look for opportunities to move your body. Many well-meaning friends and relatives try to spare older people from any exertion. It is satisfying to be able to say: "Thank you, but I'd rather do it myself. I *can*, you know."

It is always good to have some active project underway—putting in a new flower bed, cutting wood, building a fence, painting a room, mowing the lawn, and a thousand other jobs and interests that keep you busy and youthful.

KEEPING SCORE

Two of your most important pieces of fitness equipment are the pencil and paper to keep a continuous record of your status and progress. In addition to a record of your special daily exercises, you should also keep account of all other activity. Remember that the effects of exercise in some respects are cumulative, so everything you do each day counts even though it may have been gained a little at a time.

On the score card, you will note that various activities are given a point value. *Make a chart like this for yourself to use each week.*

Each day enter in the appropriate space the number of points you have earned. Activities have been grouped in several categories, and you should try to gain credits in each category.

GOALS

Add your points daily, but classify yourself according to your weekly total. As you will notice, most weekly goals allow you some time off for good (active) behavior.

Physical Activity Level	Points per Day	Points per Week
Level 1	10	70
Level 2	15	100
Level 3	20	125
Level 3+	25	150

Your total number of points should gradually increase as your physical condition improves. For example, a total of 10 points per day or 70 per week would be satisfactory for someone on Level One. The top of Level Three would give you 20 points per day or 125 per week. Once there, you can push on with an advanced schedule of activities (call it Level Three Plus) to earn 25 points per day or 150 per week. This level will keep you fairly vigorous.

These point values are approximations based upon the clinical experience of exercise specialists. It is best if you set your own goals according to the way you feel. But don't *underestimate* your vitality—and keep increasing the total points achieved each day until you become one of the "lively ones." Then stay that way.

DAILY PHYSICAL ACTIVITY SCORE CARD

In order to receive credit for the variety of activities you may participate in each day, the following classification and scoring system is given. Determine your daily physical activity score by adding up the time you spend performing various activities during the day according to categories listed below.

After adding up the approximate time spent on activities in each category, give yourself the appropriate number of points acquired in each category and total them. Do not exceed the maximum allowable points for categories 2 and 3.

	Mon	Tue	Wed	Thur	Fri	Sat	Sun	Total for week

1. Your Basic Daily Exercise Program

For performing any of the following activities, give yourself the points listed.

Level One exercise program = 5 points

Level Two exercise program = 10

Level Three exercise program = 12

Level Three + exercise program, or other programs such as Adult Physical Fitness, jogging and calisthenics, swimming, or YMCA keep-fit programs, lasting 30 minutes or more = 15–19

	Mon	Tue	Wed	Thur	Fri	Sat	Sun	Total for week

2. Light Activities

Give yourself 1 point for each hour spent in the following type activities. Maximum allowable washing, shaving

—Sitting and actively rocking, typing, writing, playing cards, peeling potatoes, polishing shoes, sewing, playing musical instrument

—Standing or slowly moving around room or yard

—Shooting pool, shuffle board

3. Light-Moderate Activities

Give yourself 2 points for each 30 minutes spent in the following type activities. Maximum allowable points per day = 8

—Domestic work—sweeping floors, ironing, washing clothes, making beds

—Light gardening, mowing lawn (power mower), washing automobile

—Light industrial work—auto repair, store clerk (not lifting), building with wood, painting, shoe repairing

—Walking on level at slow pace (2–3 mph) or down stairs

—Bicycling on level at easy pace (5½ mph)

—Canoeing slowly (2½–3 mph)

—Pitching horseshoes, playing golf with cart, archery, bowling

	Mon	Tue	Wed	Thur	Fri	Sat	Sun	Total for week

4. Moderate Activities

Give yourself 4 points for each 30 minutes spent in the following type activities. Maximum allowable points per day = 12

—Gardening—pulling weeds, digging, mowing lawn (hand mower)

—Mopping-scrubbing floor

—Walking on level briskly (3½–4 mph)

—Walking up and down small hills, in sand

—Playing Ping-Pong, golf without cart, badminton, volleyball, or tennis (doubles)

—Canoeing briskly (4 mph) or rowing for pleasure

—Dancing—fox trot, waltz, square

5. Heavy Activities

Give yourself 8 points for each 30 minutes spent in the following type activities. No maximum.

—Walking upstairs, up hills, or climbing

—Bicycling briskly or up and down hills

—Playing tennis (singles)
—Water skiing
—Cross country snow skiing
—Chopping wood, digging holes, shoveling snow

SPECIAL NOTES ON EXERCISE

Jogging

More and more people are jogging today than ever before. It is a valuable physical activity because jogging lends itself so well to gradual increase. The idea is to alternate walking and jogging bouts until you jog more than you walk. In addition, the distance covered can be gradually increased as well as the speed at which you move. The speed element, however, is not as important as getting a good workout within a reasonable time.

The walk-jog intervals outlined in the Level One, Level Two, and Level Three exercise schedules allow for easy progression. If you can handle Level Three easily and wish to go forward with jogging, by all means do so. First work up both the walking and the jogging intervals simultaneously until you are walking 100 yards and jogging 100 yards (about the length of a city block). Then hold the walking interval constant at 100 yards, but gradually increase the jogging interval to 200 yards—or more as you feel ready. Also, gradually increase the total distance covered. There are many people around the country in their sixties and seventies who are jogging two to five miles daily. But don't set your goals this high unless you have gradually raised the distances jogged without experiencing severe reactions or extreme fatigue lasting for several days. Remember, too, to "taper off" by walking the last interval and moving around until your breathing and pulse rate return to near normal.

It is important to wear the correct shoes and clothing while jogging. Clean, thick, well-fitting socks are a "must," and the shoes should also fit well and have soft, nonslip soles, with no heels. If gym shoes are worn, they should have a built-in arch support. You can buy shoes made especially for jogging. Wear loose-fitting clothes. In the winter, add a hat, ear muffs, and gloves. During the summer, you can wear a T-shirt and shorts. Summer jogging should be done either in the morning or early evening.

Jogging is great for the circulatory system and the legs but does not provide a complete and balanced workout. Therefore, calisthenics or other conditioning exercises should be added to the jogging session each day. The exercises described in this book will serve this purpose very well.

Swimming and Water Exercises

Swimming is such a good activity it deserves special mention because it involves all the major muscle groups. It can also be adjusted from a very mild to a strenuous pace, and can be easily graded for progressive conditioning by gradually increasing the distances.

You can work out your own system of interval training. For example, swim across the pool, get out and walk around to the other side and repeat this procedure until your swimming trips across total a good distance. The next progression might be to swim the length of the pool and walk back, and so on. The workout can be varied by using different strokes to swim the intervals.

The buoyancy of the water makes it easier to do some exercises. Therefore, if your physical condition is such that you cannot do even some of the Level One exercises on land, find the ones that you *can* do in the water and get your workout that way. On the other hand, the water also causes resistance for certain other exercises. Use this medium as a way of increasing the workload.

Exercise Problems Due to Foot Conditions or Leg Pains

Problems with the feet, the legs, and the knee and hip joints are fairly common. Any problems there, be it bunions, arthritic knees, or varicose veins, may interfere with proper performance of some of the exercises outlined in this book, particularly walking and jogging.

If you have such a problem, first make sure that you have done all that you can do to obtain needed medical care.

Next, do not let your problem sidetrack you in your determination to get fit. The following activities can be substituted for walking and jogging, and can provide healthful exercises.

• Swimming and water exercises.
• "Bicycling" movement, while lying on the floor, hips and legs in the air, supported by the arms and elbows. Do not try this if you think you will have difficulty supporting your weight.
• Riding a bicycle.
• Pedaling a stationary bike.
• Playing golf. (Here is one time a golf cart is justified.)
• Exercising on wall pulley-weights or rowing machine.
• Passing a medicine ball with a partner while standing or seated—or bouncing the ball off a wall in continuous rhythmic movement.

SPECIAL NOTES ON HEALTH

A program of physical fitness must, of course, include much more than exercise. It should begin with basic health considerations. Here are a few reminders:

Medical and Dental Care

The importance of periodic medical and dental checkups cannot be overemphasized. This is the best form of preventive maintenance for your body. Everyone, especially older people, should have at least an annual checkup.

If you do not have a personal physician, check on available health services with your local public health officer or the public health nurse who visits your neighborhood. If you cannot find a local public health person, ask at the closest hospital to you, or call the local medical society. Remember, it is not only important to find the physician and dentist, but it is even more necessary to follow their advice once it is given.

Remember also, your medical "advisor" should know your exercise plans before you start your program—be it Level One, Level Two, or Level Three. And let him really advise you—follow his recommendations.

Diet and Nutrition

A good basic diet is necessary at all ages and does not change radically when one approaches age sixty.

The way to good nutrition is through the four basic food groups. These groups and recommended *daily* servings are:

Bread and cereals
(4 or more servings)
Meat, poultry, fish, eggs
(2 or more servings)
Fruits and vegetables
(4 or more servings)
Dairy products
(2 or more cups of milk or its equivalent)

Overweight is a problem for many older people, and therefore the total number of calories consumed should be carefully adjusted according to individual needs. Many people become less active as they grow older, but they continue to eat the same amount of food. Because of this, they gain weight.

Older people with a very low level of energy expenditure would have to cut back their food intake severely to lose weight. But doing this would risk the loss of an adequate amount of certain vitamins and minerals necessary to good health. This is another reason for keeping active. See Chapter IX for a more complete discussion of nutrition.

Some older people find that they become uncomfortable after eating a large meal. When this happens, it may be better to spread the food intake over five or six small meals a day rather than the traditional three hearty meals. The *total* amount of food, however, should be considered in terms of daily need for calories and nutrients.

Sleep and Rest

As you grow older, you may need more sleep or rest. The day's program should include rest periods. A nap in the afternoon is probably a good idea. Several rest periods or "cat naps" are particularly desirable for the person who usually sleeps less than eight hours during the night.

Cigarette Smoking

Cigarette smoking has been linked to lung cancer, emphysema (a serious lung condition that makes breathing difficult), bronchitis, and heart disease. The data show that the chances of developing these chronic diseases are related to the number of years a person has been smoking as well as the number of cigarettes smoked. The evidence also indicates that it is possible to overcome some of the harmful effects. That is, the sooner a smoker stops and the longer he stays stopped, the better his chances of improved health.

Cigars and pipes seem to be less harmful than cigarettes for the heart and lungs. There is, however, a higher rate of lip and mouth cancer among cigar and pipe smokers.

The facts call out loudly, "If you smoke, stop; if you do not smoke, do not start." By increasing the amount of your daily exercise, you can prevent the weight increase that some people experience when they stop smoking.

So, That's the Challenge

The exercises are here. Now the rest is up to you. It will not be easy to get going, especially if you have not been active for a long time. There is no easy way to fitness. But once you get started, you will begin to feel the benefits and, before long, you will be looking forward to your daily exercise. The self-discipline you must use pays off in two ways: You keep boredom at a minimum, and you live a more zestful and worthwhile life.

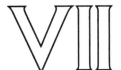

Exercises
for
Teenagers

Your teen years are busy years. There is your school work and your social life. But with all this activity, it is still important to develop a regular program of exercise. An alert mind, so necessary for good grades, is dependent, in part, on a healthy body. And, too, so many of your other activities—club work, an after-school job, parties and dances—require stamina. A good physical fitness program will help you maintain a high energy level. If you are already in good shape, you will be able to enjoy these carefree years more fully and still stay in good shape.

During the teen years, physical activity usually begins to slow down. Certainly there is more school work to be done, which leaves less time for relaxation, but this is not the only reason for the decrease. A lot of time is spent chatting with friends either on the telephone or over a soda at a snack bar. Movie-going and television-watching take up their share of time, too. And a driver's license usually comes into the picture. Once a teen has access to a car, walking and bike riding become activities of the past. The novelty of driving is too strong a pull.

While the amount of physical activity tends to decrease, the caloric intake tends to increase. A teenager's favorite meal seems to be a hamburger and french fries washed down by a soft drink or a shake. No wonder many young adults trace their weight problems to their high school years.

Rather than face a flabby future, why not get into the exercise habit right now? Make daily physical activity as automatic as brushing your teeth. Set aside at least thirty minutes a day for exercise. It is an investment that will pay high dividends in the future.

PHYSICAL FITNESS REQUIRES PHYSICAL CARE

Make a point of having a physical checkup at least once a year, and see your dentist at least twice a year. You now have the only set of natural teeth that you will ever have. With good care, your teeth will last, and you can avoid the nuisance of dentures in your later years.

While you are in high school, many of your friends may claim it is "adult" to smoke, drink, or use drugs. Tobacco, alcohol, and drugs will do your body no good. Exercise and a sound diet, on the other hand, will never hurt you.

WHAT THIS PROGRAM IS ALL ABOUT

These exercises are designed for teenagers who are not active in sports programs. Many teens, of course, play on their school teams. If you are a member of a sports team, you may be in excellent physical condition already. These exercises, though, will help you stay in shape during the off-season.

This program is designed to develop your:

1. Cardiovascular endurance
2. Arm and shoulder strength
3. Abdominal strength
4. Agility

A word of caution: You should never begin any exercise program, including this one, without first checking with your doctor. Chances are that a physical checkup will show that you can follow this program without endangering your health.

While doing these exercises, if you experience any of these symptoms, stop immediately and do not continue with the program until you have talked with your doctor:

1. Excessive breathlessness. Some breathlessness is normal with exercise. You should, though, return to your normal rate of breathing soon after you stop exercising.

2. Blue lips and/or nails. Unless you are exercising in cold, damp air, your lips and nails should not turn blue.

3. Cold sweat.

4. Unusual fatigue. If you are not in topnotch physical condition, you will be tired after exercise, but you should not be worn out or exhausted.

5. Persistent shakiness. Any shakiness that lasts for more than ten minutes is persistent.

6. Muscle twitching. We all have a twitching muscle occasionally, but it should not happen after every exercise session.

You should also check with your doctor if you experience these symptoms on a *regular* basis:

1. Headache
2. Dizziness
3. Fainting
4. Broken sleep
5. Digestive upset
6. Pain not resulting from an injury
7. Undue pounding or uneven heartbeat
8. Disorientation or personality changes

While all of these symptoms may simply mean that you are physically unfit, only your doctor can tell for certain. Rather than take unnecessary chances, check with him.

BEFORE YOU START: THE RECOVERY INDEX TEST

You will have to find out how you respond to exercise that is moderately strenuous. The Recovery Index Test is one way to find out. All you have to do is step up and down a platform thirty times in one minute for four minutes. The platform should be at least fourteen inches high but no more than twenty inches. You decide what is the most comfortable height for you.

If possible, have someone else keep time

for you. When you take this test alone, use a clock with a second hand. To take the test, count one and place one foot on the platform, then the other. Step down, one foot at a time. On the count of two, repeat the action. At the end of four minutes, you should have stepped up and down the platform 120 times. Now take your pulse according to the following schedule:

1. One minute after the exercise for 30 seconds.
2. Two minutes after the exercise for 30 seconds.
3. Three minutes after the exercise for 30 seconds.

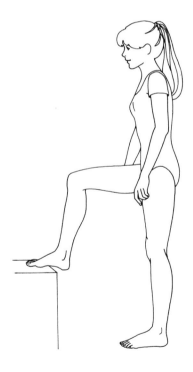

To take your pulse, turn one hand palm up. Place the fingers of your other hand on your wrist and count the pulse for thirty seconds. After you have taken your pulse three times, add up the rates to get your Recovery Index and check it against this chart:

When the three 30-second pulse counts total:	The Recovery Index is:	Then the response to this test is:
199 or more	60 or less	Poor
from 171 to 198	between 61 and 70	Fair
from 150 to 170	between 71 and 80	Good
from 133 to 149	between 81 and 90	Very Good
132 or less	91 or more	Excellent

As you progress with your exercise program, give yourself a Recovery Index Test at least once a month. Unless you are already in top shape, you should see a gradual improvement in your recovery rate. This test, however, is not meant to determine your overall fitness; it merely gauges your recovery after a slightly strenuous activity.

FURTHER FITNESS TESTS

FLEXED-ARM HANG (GIRLS)
Arm and Shoulder Strength

Equipment: For this test, you will need a sturdy bar adjusted to equal your height. If a bar is not available, skip this test.

Starting Position: Using an overhand grip, hang with chin above bar and elbows flexed. Legs must be straight and feet off the floor.

Action: Hold position as long as possible.

Rules: Timing should start as soon as you are in position. Timing should stop when your chin touches or drops below the bar. Do not bend your knees or kick your legs.

To Pass: If you are thirteen to seventeen years old, you should hold for three seconds.

PULL-UPS (BOYS)
Arm and Shoulder Strength

Equipment: A bar of sufficient height, comfortable to grip.

Starting Position: Grasp the bar with palms facing forward; hang with arms and legs fully extended. Feet must be free of floor.

Action: Count 1. Pull your body up with the arms until the chin is higher than bar.

Count 2. Lower your body until arms are fully extended.

Repeat as many times as possible.

Rules: The pull-up must be smooth, not a snap movement, legs must be kept straight and not kicked. One pull-up is counted each time you raise your chin above the bar.

To Pass: AGES
13—1 pull-up
14—2 pull-ups
15—3 pull-ups
16—4 pull-ups
17—5 pull-ups

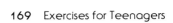

SIT-UPS (BOYS AND GIRLS)
Abdominal Strength

Do this exercise on a soft surface such as a rug or a mat.

Starting Position: Lie on your back with knees flexed, feet about one foot apart. Your hands, with fingers laced, are behind your head. Have someone hold your ankles to keep your feet on the floor.

Action: Count 1. Sit up and turn your body to the left, touching your right elbow to your left knee.

Count 2. Return to starting position.

Count 3. Sit up and turn your body to the right, touching your left elbow to your right knee.

Count 4. Return to starting position. Repeat as many times as you can. Each time you return to the starting position, you have completed one sit-up.

To Pass:

AGES	GIRLS	BOYS
13	20	38
14	20	45
15	20	49
16	20	50
17	20	50

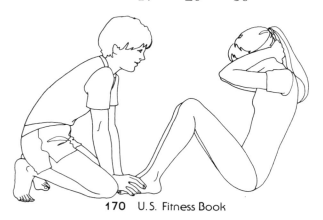

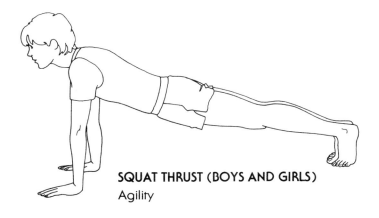

SQUAT THRUST (BOYS AND GIRLS)
Agility

Have someone keep time for you. Do as many squat thrusts as you can in ten seconds.

Starting Position: Stand erect.

Action: Count 1. Bend knees and place hands on floor in front of feet. Arms may be between, outside or in front of knees.

Count 2. Thrust legs back until the body is perfectly straight from shoulders to feet (pushup position).

Count 3. Return to squat position.

Count 4. Return to standing position.

To Pass: GIRLS
AGES
13–17—3 squat thrusts in ten seconds
BOYS
AGES
13–17—4 squat thrusts in ten seconds

YOUR EXERCISE PROGRAM

These exercises, unless otherwise marked, are for both boys and girls. The calisthenic exercises are arranged in order of difficulty. The easiest, a warm-up exercise, comes first. The other exercises are progressively more difficult. Each day, before starting your exercises, do the warm-up.

The first week or two of your exercise program should be devoted to learning the exercises. Once you have mastered them, start out slowly, doing each one three to five times, working up to ten. You will, of course, not be able to do all the exercises in a thirty-minute or so period. Go in a cycle. For instance, let us assume that on Monday you do the first ten exercises, excluding the warm-up, ten times each. On Tuesday then, you begin with the eleventh exercise and so on. When you have worked your way through all the exercises, simply start the cycle over.

As your level of fitness improves, you will find that you can accomplish more and more in the thirty-minute period.

A Tip: You may find that doing your exercises to music helps you establish a rhythm. At the beginning, though, select a slow tempo.

DEEP BREATHER
Warm-up—Respiratory System

Starting Position: Stand at attention.

Action: Count 1. Rise on toes while circling the arms inward and upward slowly, and inhaling deeply. At the end of movement, arms are extended overhead.

Count 2. Continue circling arms backward and downward while lowering the heels and exhaling.

This exercise should be done slowly and rhythmically.

WING STRETCHER
Flexibility—Back and Chest

Starting Position: Stand erect; raise elbows to shoulder height, fists clenched, palms down in front of chest.
Action: Thrust elbows backward vigorously and return. Be sure head remains erect. Keep elbows at shoulder height.

ONE-FOOT BALANCE
Balance

Starting Position: Stand at attention.
Action: Count 1. Stretch left leg backward, while bending trunk forward and extending arms sideward until this position is reached: The head is up, trunk parallel to floor; the left leg is fully extended with toes of left foot pointed. The supporting leg is kept straight. Hold this position for 5 to 10 seconds. Return to starting position.
Count 2. Repeat, using the opposite leg for support.

JUMPING JACK
Coordination—Cardiovascular

Starting Position: Stand at attention.
Action: Count 1. Swing arms sideward and upward,

touching hands above head (arms straight) while simultaneously moving feet sideward and apart in a single jumping motion.

Count 2. Spring back to the starting position.

BODY BENDER
Flexibility—Lateral Trunk

Starting Position: Stand, feet slightly apart, hands clasped behind the head.

Action: Count 1. Bend sideward at the hips to the left as far as possible. Keep the feet stationary and the toes pointed straight ahead.

Count 2. Return to starting position.

Count 3. Repeat, bending to the right.

Count 4. Return to the starting position.

WINDMILL
Flexibility—Lower Back, Hamstrings

Starting Position: Stand, knees flexed, feet spread shoulder width apart, arms extended sideward shoulder-high, palms down.

Action: Count 1. Twist and bend trunk, bringing right hand to the left toe, keeping arms straight, knees flexed.

Count 2. Return to starting position.

Count 3. Twist and bend trunk, bringing left hand to the right toe, keeping arms straight, knees flexed.

Count 4. Return to starting position.

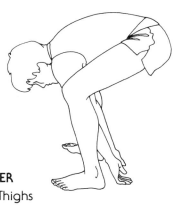

BACK STRETCHER
Lower Back—Thighs

Starting Position: Stand with feet spread apart, arms extended overhead.

Action: Count 1. Bend forward from hips, knees bent. Swing arms downward between legs. Count 2. Return to starting position.

JUMP AND TOUCH
Leg Extensors

Starting Position: Assume a half-crouch position, bending from the waist as though about to begin a broad jump. Arms are extended backward.

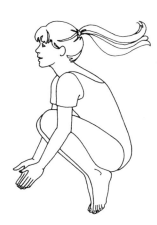

Action: Spring straight upward, bringing knees to the chest and heels to buttocks, meanwhile swinging the arms downward and around the legs, attempting to touch hands together under the legs. Land in the starting position, ready for the next upward leap.

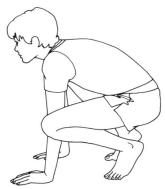

SQUAT THRUST
Cardiovascular—Agility

Starting Position: Stand at attention.

Action: Count 1. Bend knees and place hands on the floor in front of the feet. Arms may be between, outside of, or in front of the bent knees.

Count 2. Thrust the legs back far enough so that the body is perfectly straight from shoulders to feet (the pushup position).

Count 3. Return to squat position.

Count 4. Return to erect position.

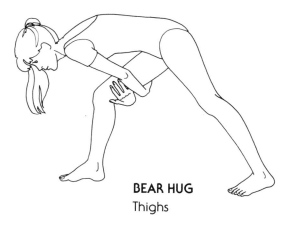

BEAR HUG
Thighs

Starting Position: Stand, feet comfortably spread, with hands on hips.

Action: Count 1. Take a long step diagonally right, keeping left foot anchored in place; tackle the right leg around the thigh by encircling the thigh with both arms.

Count 2. Return to the starting position.

Counts 3 and 4. Repeat to the opposite side.

THE COORDINATOR

Coordination—Cardiovascular

Starting Position: Stand at attention.

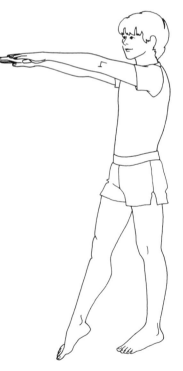

Action: Count 1. Hop on left foot, swinging right leg forward, touching toe to floor in front of left foot, meanwhile bringing both arms forward to shoulder level, fully extended.

Count 2. Hop again on left foot, swinging right foot to the right side and touching toe to floor, meanwhile flinging arms sideward at shoulder level.

Count 3. Hop again on left foot, returning to position of Count 1.

Count 4. Hop again on left foot, returning to starting position.

Repeat, hopping on right foot. Continue, alternately hopping on each foot. As exercise is mastered, tempo should be increased.

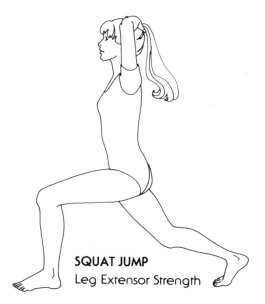

SQUAT JUMP
Leg Extensor Strength

Starting Position: Assume semi-squat position, hands clasped on top of head, feet apart, heel of left foot on line with toes of the right foot.

Action: Count 1. Spring upward from the floor, reversing the position of the feet and coming down to the semi-squat position. Hands remain on head.

Count 2. Same movement, reversing feet.

Continue, reversing feet on each upward jump.

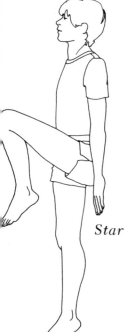

KNEE RAISE (SINGLE AND DOUBLE)
Hip Flexors and Abdominals

Starting Position: Lie on back with knees slightly flexed, feet on floor, arms at side.

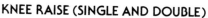

Action: Count 1. Raise one knee up as close as possible to chest.

Count 2. Fully extend the knee so the leg is perpendicular to the floor.

Count 3. Bend knee and return to chest.

Count 4. Straighten leg and return to starting position.

Alternate the legs during the exercise. The double knee raise is done in the same manner by moving both legs simultaneously.

HEAD AND SHOULDER CURL
Abdominals and Hip Flexors

Starting Position: Lie on back with hands at sides, palms down.

Action: Count 1. Lift the head and shoulders off the floor. Hold the tense position for four counts.

Count 2. Return to starting position.

LEG EXTENSION
Hip Flexors and Abdominals

Starting Position: Sit, legs extended, body erect and hands on hips.

Action: Count 1. With a quick, vigorous action, raise and flex the knees by dragging feet backward toward the buttocks with the toes lightly touching the ground.

Count 2. Extend the legs back to the starting position.

The head and shoulders should be held high throughout the exercise.

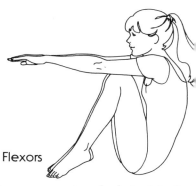

UP OARS
Abdominals and Hip Flexors

Starting Position: Lie on back with arms extended behind head.

Action: Count 1. Sit up, reach forward with the extended arms, meanwhile pulling the knees tightly against the chest. Arms are outside the knees.

Count 2. Return to starting position. The exercise is done rhythmically and without breaks in the movement.

SNAP AND TWIST
Abdominal and Hip Flexors

Starting Position: Lie on back with arms extended beyond head.

Action: Count 1. With a vigorous action, sit up and bring the left knee to chest while extending right arm forward and the left elbow backward. (This is an explosive type of movement.)

Count 2. Return to the starting position.

Count 3. Repeat the movement to the opposite side.

Count 4. Return to starting position. The exercise is done rhythmically.

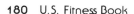

BACK TWIST
Hip Flexors and Abdominals

Starting Position: Lie on back, arms extended sideward, palms on the floor, and legs raised to a vertical position.

Action: Count 1. Keeping both feet together, swing legs slowly to the left until almost touching the floor. Keep arms, shoulders, and head in contact with the floor.
Count 2. Return to starting position.
Count 3. Repeat the movement to the right.
Count 4. Return to starting position.

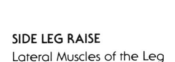

SIDE LEG RAISE
Lateral Muscles of the Leg

Starting Position: Lie on side, arms extended overhead. The head rests on the lower arm. Legs are extended fully, one on top of the other.

Action: Count 1. With a brisk action, raise the top leg vertically.
Count 2. Return to starting position. Repeat for specified number of counts and repeat on other side.

THE SPRINTER
Cardiovascular, Arms and Legs

Starting Position: Assume squatting position, hands on the floor, fingers pointed forward, left leg fully extended to the rear.

Action: Count 1. Reverse position of the feet by bringing left foot to hands and extending right leg backward, all in one motion.

Count 2. Reverse feet again, returning to starting position.

Repeat exercise rhythmically.

PUSH-UPS
Arms, Shoulders and Chest Muscles

Starting Position: Boys: Extend arms and place hands on ground just under and slightly outside of the shoulders, fingers pointing forward. Extend body so that it is perfectly straight. The weight is supported on the hands and toes. Girls: Extend arms and place hands, fingers pointing forward, on ground just under and slightly outside of the shoulders. Place knees on floor and extend body until it is straight from the head to the knees. Bend knees and raise the feet off the floor. The weight is supported by the hands and knees. (Also for boys who cannot do regular push-ups.)

Action: Count 1. Keeping body tense and straight, bend elbows and touch chest to floor.

Count 2. Return to original position. (The body must be kept perfectly straight. The buttocks must not be raised. The abdomen must not sag.)

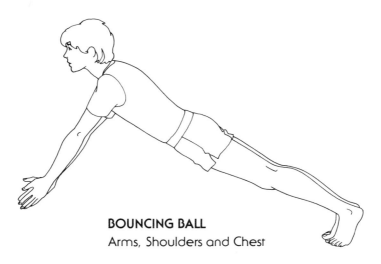

BOUNCING BALL
Arms, Shoulders and Chest

Starting Position: Assume push-up position, by bending forward, extending the arms and placing the hands on the floor, shoulder width apart, fingers pointing forward, and extending trunk and legs backward in a straight line. The body is supported on the hands and toes.

Action: Bounce up and down by a series of short, upward springs. (Try clapping hands together while body is in the air.)

SOME ALTERNATIVE EXERCISES

You can vary your exercise program with these activities. Just give yourself plenty of room; better yet, do them out of doors.

All Fours. Face down, on hands and feet. Walk forward.

Bear Walk. Face down, on hands and feet, travel forward by moving the right arm and right leg simultaneously, and then the left arm and left leg simultaneously.

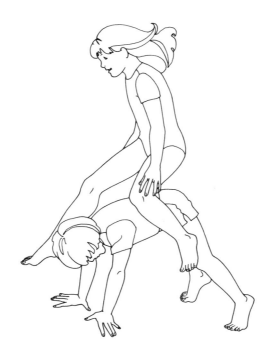

Leap Frog. Count off by twos. On command, the "evens" leap over the "odds." At the next command the "odds" leap over the "evens."

Indian Walk. Bend knees slightly, bend trunk forward, arms hanging down until backs of hands touch the ground. Retain this position and walk forward.

Crouch Run. Lean forward at the waist until the trunk is parallel with the ground. Retain this position and run slowly.

Straddle Run. Run forward, leaping obliquely to the right as the right foot advances, leaping obliquely to the left as the left foot advances.

Knee-Raised Run. Run forward, raising the knees as high as possible on each step. Pump arms vigorously.

One-Leg Hop. Travel forward by hopping on the left foot. Take long steps. Change to right foot and repeat.

As a high school student, you are no doubt taking a course of physical education. This allows you other opportunities for exercise. You can learn to use exercise apparatus such as ropes and parallel bars. You can also do tumbling and weight lifting. By the way, there is no reason why girls cannot work with weights and barbells; they will not become muscle-bound. If your school does not offer any of these activities, perhaps a local youth organization does. Do not, however, take up these activities on your own. You must be taught by a qualified instructor. Unless you have proper training in using exercise apparatus or in tumbling and weight lifting, you risk injury.

JOGGING

Jogging is not only great exercise, but it is also very popular. Regular jogging can condition your heart to work more but with less effort; increase the efficiency of your respiratory system; increase the blood volume of your body; keep your blood vessels flexible; aid your digestive system; and keep your weight down.

How to Jog

Run in an upright position and avoid the tendency to lean. Keep your back as straight as you can and still remain comfortable. Keep your head up and do not look at your feet.

Hold your arms slightly away from your body and bend your elbows so that your forearms are approximately parallel to the ground. Occasionally shake your arms and relax your shoulders to avoid the tightness that sometimes occurs while jogging. Periodically, take several deep breaths and blow them out completely. This will help you relax.

If you can, start each step on the heel of your foot and end on the ball. Should this be uncomfortable, jog in a more flat-footed style. Do not jog on the balls of your feet as though you were sprinting. Using only the balls of your feet can make your legs very sore.

Keep your steps short, letting your foot strike the ground beneath your knee. The length of your stride should vary with your rate of speed. Breathe deeply, with your mouth open. Do not hold your breath.

If for any reason you become unusually tired or uncomfortable, slow down, walk, or stop.

What to Wear

Select loose, comfortable clothes. Dress for warmth in the winter, for coolness in the summer. Avoid tight clothing which restricts your freedom of movement. "Jogging suits" or "warm-ups" are not necessary, but they are extremely practical and comfortable.

Do not wear rubberized or plastic clothing. Increased sweating will not produce permanent weight loss, but it can cause body temperature to rise to dangerous levels. It interferes with sweat evaporation, the body's chief temperature-control mechanism during exercise. If sweat cannot evaporate, heat stroke or heat exhaustion can result.

Properly fitting shoes with firm soles, good arch supports and pliable tops are essential. Shoes made especially for distance running or walking are recommended. Ripple or crepe soles are excellent for running on hard surfaces. Beginners should avoid inexpensive, thin-soled sneakers. Wear clean, soft, heavy, well-fitting socks. Beginners may want to wear thin socks under the heavier pair.

Where to Jog

If possible, avoid hard surfaces such as concrete and asphalt for the first few weeks. Running tracks (located at most high schools), grass playing fields, parks and golf courses are recommended. In bad weather, jog in church, school or YMCA gymnasiums; in protected areas around shopping centers; or in your garage or basement. Varying locations and routes will add interest to your program.

When to Jog

The time of day is not important. It is best not to jog during the first half hour after eating, or during a hot, humid day. The important thing is to commit yourself to a regular schedule. Studies show that people who jog early in the morning tend to be more faithful than those who run in the evenings. People who jog with family members or friends also tend to keep to their schedules better. However, companionship, not competition, should be your goal when jogging with someone else.

Illness or Injuries

Take care to prevent blisters, sore muscles and aching joints. If you develop an illness, ask your physician if you should keep jogging. Any persistent pain or soreness also should be reported.

The following sample training schedules are recommended. Each X represents one execution of the given distance (e.g., in week 1, jog 440 yards twice and 660 yards three times each day.

GIRLS' TWELVE-WEEK JOGGING SCHEDULE

Distance	1	2	3	4	5	6	7	8	9	10	11	12
440 yards	XX	XX	X	X								
660 yards	XXX	XX	XX	X	X	X	X					
880 yards		X	XX	X	XX	X	X	X	X	X	X	X
1100 yards				XX	X	XX	X	X	XX	X	X	X
1320 yards					X	X	XX	X	X	X	X	X
1 mile								XX	X	X	X	X
1¼ mile										X	X	X

BOYS' TWELVE-WEEK JOGGING SCHEDULE

Distance	1	2	3	4	5	6	7	8	9	10	11	12
660 yards	XX	XX	X	X								
880 yards	XXX	XX	XX	X	X	X	X					
1320 yards		X	XX	X	XX	X	X	X	X	X	X	X
1 mile				XX	X	XX	X	X	X	X	X	X
1¼ mile					X	X	XX	X	XX	X	X	X
1½ mile								XX	X	X	X	X
1¾ mile										X	X	X

GOOD POSTURE

Good posture is important to good health and appearance. Slouching is not only unattractive, but it also puts pressure on your internal organs. Usually it is the abdominal organs such as the stomach that suffer most from poor posture. When the body is carried in a sloppy way, the bones are out of line and the muscles take unnecessary strain. Quite often a feeling of tiredness results.

Holding your body properly promotes good health and projects a poised, confident image. Why not get into the habit of good posture?

Front View of Good Posture

Hold your head erect.

Keep your shoulders level.

Let your arms hang easily at your sides with the palms of your hands toward your body.

Keep your hips level, and your weight supported equally by both legs.

Keep your kneecaps facing straight ahead.

Keep your feet pointed straight ahead.

The weight of your body should be carried toward the outer sides of your feet and be evenly balanced between the heel and the forefoot.

Good posture is built from the feet up. If your feet and knees are in good position, there is a better chance that the rest of your body will line up as it should.

Back View of Good Posture

Your head is straight.

Your shoulders are level.

Your shoulder blades are flat against your upper back, not protruding or winged and not far apart or squeezed close together.

Your arms hang easily at your sides, your palms are toward your body.

Your spine is straight.

Your hips are level, and your weight is supported equally by both legs.

Your legs are straight.

Your heel cords are straight.

Side View of Good Posture

Your head is erect. Your chin is above the notch between your collar bones, with a slight forward curve in your neck.

Your shoulders are in line with your ears.

Your arm hangs easily at your side.

Your upper back is erect.

Your chest is slightly elevated because your upper back is erect.

Your abdominal wall is flat.

Your lower back is held in good position (curved slightly forward).

Your hips are midway between forward and backward tilt.

Your knees are straight but "easy." They are not bent, pushed back, or stiff.

Your feet are pointed straight ahead. Your weight is carried over the arch, evenly balanced between the heel and the forefoot.

Posture in Sitting

To sit erect and be at ease, the type and size of the chair must be suited to the individual. A person can rest back against a straight-back chair and be in good posture.

Sitting "slumped" puts a strain on many parts of the body, especially the back. (Besides, it puts a strain on the people who have to look at you!)

Sitting up too straight arches the lower back too much. A person cannot sit at ease in this position.

Let your posture in sitting be graceful, never disgraceful!

Sit with your knees together and your feet flat on the floor, or with feet crossed, or at times with your knees crossed. If your knees are crossed, one over the other, they should be alternated so they are not always crossed in the same manner.

While some people, especially those with problems of poor circulation in the legs, should avoid sitting with their knees crossed, there is good reason why so many people sit this way. Unless a person is sitting in a chair that gives adequate support to the lower back, there is a tendency, when one tries to sit erect, for the hips to tilt forward to the point of arching the lower back. If the knees are crossed, the hips cannot tilt as far forward, and the hips and lower back are in a more stable position.

Descriptive Comments to Help Promote and Maintain Good Posture

• Stand tall. Remember that the tallest distance between your head and your hips is a straight spine, but slight curves are normal. To check for normal curves of your spine, stand with your back to a wall, heels about 2 inches from the wall. Place one hand behind your neck with the back of the hand against the wall, and the other hand behind your lower back with the palm against the wall. Now your entire back should touch either your hands or the wall.

• Let your arms hang easily at your sides as you draw your shoulder blades back. Do not push your elbows back beyond the side line of the body.

• The position of your hips controls the position of your lower back. Keep your hips midway between a forward tilt and a backward tilt to maintain the normal curve in your lower back. Belts on trousers or skirts should be parallel with the ground.

• The position of your upper back controls the position of your neck. Your head tends to stay level (because eyes seek eye-level) but if the upper back slumps your neck curves forward. If the upper back is straightened, the curve in the neck tends to return to normal.

• The position of your upper back also controls the position of your chest. As you straighten your upper back, your chest is raised into good position. Do *not* try to bring your chest up by arching your lower back. It *must* be done by your upper back.

• Place weight evenly on both feet.

• Keep both your knees straight, not bent or pushed back.

• Stand in front of a mirror and try to make your hips level and shoulders level.

A FINAL WORD

You now have a solid program of physical fitness. One that will serve you well if you use it. There is nothing wrong with having pride in your body, in wanting to stay fit and healthy. Indeed, it is a sign of maturity to assume care of your body. Here's to the best years of your life!

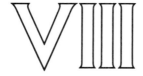

Children's Exercises

Everyone needs exercise, and that includes small children, those who have learned to walk. Infants, of course, provide their own exercise by just waving their arms and kicking their legs. If your child is still a "crawler," all you have to do is allow a safe place for the child. Then let the youngster crawl. When the weather permits, a crawl session outside is a fine idea.

For the toddler, a short walk whenever possible is all the exercise you need provide. As any parent knows, small children give themselves more than enough exercise. Once your child is really up and walking, from about three on, it is time to think about regular daily exercise.

The most important thing you can do to encourage good physical habits in your child is to avoid the temptation to use the television set as an electronic babysitter. Whenever the weather permits, urge your child to play outside. If you can, invest in a sturdy swing set and then let the child use it often. Where a swing set is not feasible, take your child to a nearby park or playground for an hour or so every day. Walk there and back if the distance is not too great.

Another fine exercise aid is a tricycle (and later a bicycle) or any toy that requires pedaling. As soon as your child is old enough, buy one. Always encourage safe running, jumping, and climbing games such as tag, hide-and-seek, and jump rope.

If you decide to enroll your child in a day-care center, ask about the physical activities. A good day-care program will include some form of exercise. When your child is left in the care of a daily sitter, insist on regular daily outside play.

When your child starts school, remember there is no need to drive him or her to a bus stop only a few short blocks away. Walking is good exercise at any age.

As your child grows older and begins to display interest in team sports, encourage the interest. This does not mean that you have to pay for private tennis lessons or build a swimming pool. Lessons, where necessary, do not have to be private or expensive. Check into the various programs offered by such organizations as the YMCA. A child can often get lessons at low cost. Just show a sincere interest in what your child is doing, give generous praise, and provide whatever equipment you can. Take an interest, too, in the physical education program offered at your child's school.

But, above all, remember that children are great little imitators. If your child sees you

exercising regularly, he or she will want t
join in.

DO'S AND DON'TS FOR PARENTS

- DO teach your child the rules of safety.
- DO encourage your child to develo good posture habits.
- DO take your child for regular medica and dental examinations.
- DO check with your physician if an problems develop when starting you child on any exercise or sports activity
- DO NOT compare your child's perfor mance with that of another child.
- DO NOT force your child into any gam or exercise.

WARNING SIGNS

If your child displays any of these symptom during play or exercise, consult with you physician immediately.

Excessive breathlessness. Some breath lessness is normal after any vigorous activity but the child should return to a normal rat of breathing in two or three minutes.

Blue lips or nailbeds. Unless the child i playing in cold, damp air, this should no happen.

Cold sweat. This is rarely, if ever, a norma reaction.

Unusual fatigue. If you notice this, do no assume that your child is being lazy.

Shakiness. There may be some shakines

after vigorous play, but it should not last more than ten minutes.

Muscle twitching. If you notice that your child develops twitching each time he or she plays or exercises, check into it.

Occasionally children also exhibit the following symptoms. So long as they are only *occasional,* you probably have no cause for alarm. If they persist, however, check with your physician.

1. Headache
2. Dizziness
3. Fainting
4. Broken night's sleep
5. Digestive upset
6. Pain not associated with an injury
7. Unusual pounding or uneven heartbeat
8. Disorientation or personality changes

HE EXERCISES

The following exercises are simple and easy to learn. They are not, however, meant for children younger than six. It is also wise for these exercises to be done with an adult close by. With older children, say from ten on, supervision may not be necessary.

WHEELBARROW
Arm, Shoulder and Abdominal Strength

Starting Position: This is an exercise for two children. One kneels on the floor and places hands flat, di-

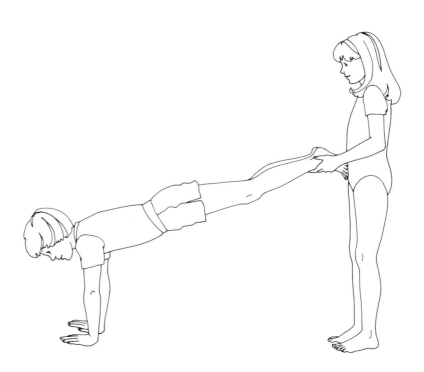

rectly under the shoulders, fingers pointing
forward. The other grasps the kneeling
child's ankles and raises the legs.

Action: The first child walks forward on the hands
feet and legs supported by partner walking
between the outstretched legs. The child
should walk three feet.

TORTOISE AND HARE: RUNNING IN PLACE
Cardiovascular

Starting Position: Child stands at attention.
Action: Count 1. Jog slowly in place.
Count 2. On the command, "Hare," the
tempo doubles. The knees are lifted high.
while arms pump vigorously.
Count 3. On the command, "Tortoise," the

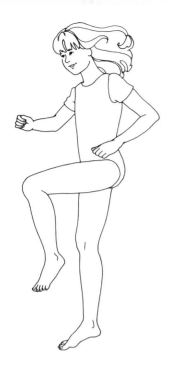

tempo slows to an easy jog. Repeat the commands, "Tortoise," "Hare." Maintain each tempo for one minute. Entire exercise time is four minutes.

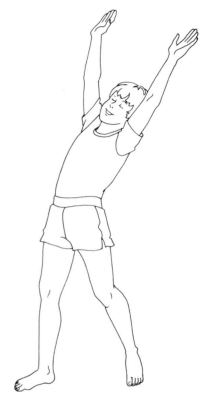

TREES IN THE WIND
Flexibility—Lateral Trunk

Starting Position: Children stand in position to move around in a circle, with arms raised and extended overhead.

Action: Children run slowly around in a circle, bending left, right, forward and back as though they were swaying in the breeze. Maintain for three or four minutes.

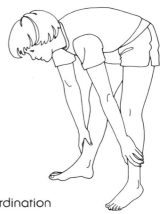

GORILLA WALK
Flexibility and Coordination

Starting Position: Child spreads feet shoulder width, bends at the waist, and grasps ankles, keeping the knees fully extended.

Action: Walk forward holding firmly to the ankles. Keep the knees extended and the legs straight. The child should go three feet.

BUNNY HOP
Leg Extensors

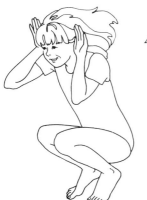

Starting Position: Child assumes squat position, ready to move around in a circle, with hands behind ears, palms forward, to simulate rabbit ears.

Action: Child moves around in a circle by hopping with both feet together, landing in the squat position. This should last for two minutes.

HOP
Leg Extensors

Starting Position: Child stands straight.

Action: Child moves forward by hopping on the left foot, taking several long steps.

Repeat, hopping on right foot. The child moves forward three feet on each foot.

BEAR WALK
Flexibility—Hamstrings

Starting Position: Child bends forward from the waist and places hands on the floor.

Action: Child moves around in a circle, moving right arm and right leg simultaneously as one step, then left arm and left leg. The child should make four circles.

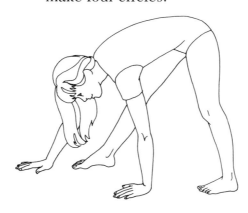

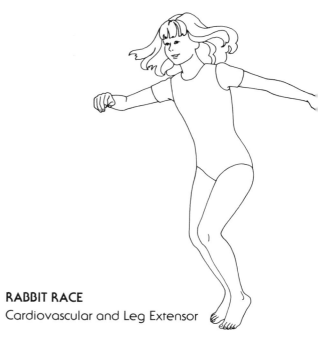

RABBIT RACE
Cardiovascular and Leg Extensor

Starting Position: This is an exercise for two or more children. Children stand in a straight line side by side, 3 feet apart. A finish line is designated 60 feet in front of the children.

Action: Children race by hopping with both feet together—first to the right, then to the left, then straight ahead, repeating this pattern until reaching the finish line.

The race may be varied by hopping in other ways—on one leg, for instance.

KNEE DOWN
Leg Extensor Strength and Balance

Starting Position: Child stands with toes of both feet on a line.

Action: Without using the hands or moving the toes from the line, kneel on both knees. Return to standing position without using hands and keeping toes on the line. Repeat five times.

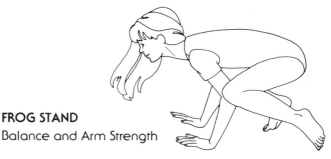

FROG STAND
Balance and Arm Strength

Starting Position: Child assumes squat position, hands on floor, fingers pointing forward. The elbows are inside of, and pressed against, knees.

Action: Lean forward slowly, transferring body weight to hands, raising feet clear of the floor. Maintain balance, keeping head up. Hold for several seconds, then return to starting position. Repeat, maintaining balance for increasingly longer periods.

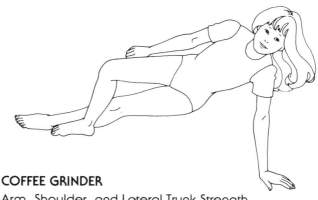

COFFEE GRINDER
Arm, Shoulder, and Lateral Trunk Strength

Starting Position: Child supports extended body (turned sideward) on right arm and both feet. Right arm and both legs are fully extended, feet slightly apart.

Action: Move feet and body in a circle, using the right arm as a pivot. Repeat, using the left arm.

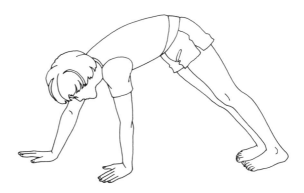

MEASURING WORM

Flexibility—Lower Back and Hamstrings

Starting Position: Child assumes the push-up position, body extended, face down, arms extended fully, shoulder width apart, hands on floor, fingers spread and pointed forward. The body is supported on hands and toes.

Action: Hold the hands stationary and walk feet up, as close to the hands as possible. Then, keeping the feet stationary, walk hands forward to starting position. Repeat alternate actions five times each.

A FINAL WORD

Exercise should never be presented as a "chore." Rather it should be kept on an informal level. You might also consider sharing exercise time with your child. Set aside time each day when you and your child do exercises together.

But however you arrange an exercise program for your child, you will be giving the youngster a priceless gift—a strong, healthy body.

Nutrition for Fitness

Anybody can maintain his weight if his energy intake (food) equals his energy output (exercise). This is true for everyone, no matter what age or sex. So long as you burn up the calories you get from your daily food, your weight will stay about the same. When you eat more food than your body needs, you gain weight.

Over the years, people have tried to lose weight by cutting down on their daily caloric intake. For some people, losing weight is simply a matter of exercising more. For others, losing weight is a combination of reduced food intake and increased exercise. Just "cutting down on calories" is a slow way to lose weight. Even when we eat less, we still tend to eat more than we need.

Actually, the lack of regular exercise is usually the cause of "creeping obesity." Because of our mechanized society, very few people have jobs that call for vigorous activity. Despite the fact that we have more free time available, most people prefer to relax by not moving around. According to recent studies, there would be fewer weight problems in this country if we exercised more.

No matter whether you are underweight, overweight, or just right, exercise and sensible eating are important to you. Only a physician, however, can determine what your weight should be. If you are too thin or too heavy, your doctor can recommend a healthy diet for you. Quite often, people make false assumptions about their weight. Some people feel they have to lose weight when indeed they should gain a bit. Others feel they are not overweight when they are. Very few people can be objective about their weight. This is one reason why you should ask your doctor's opinion.

Weight-Control Fallacies

Many people believe that it takes a great deal of time and effort to correct a weight problem. They also believe that exercise increases their appetite, causing them to eat more and gain weight. Scientific research on animals and humans has proved that these beliefs are fallacies.

Facts about Weight

1. In most people, fat piles up by only a few calories a day.
2. An excess of only 100 calories a day can

produce a ten-pound gain in a year. These extra calories could be burned up by a fifteen- or twenty-minute walk each day.

3. Overweight people are usually less active than those who are not.

4. If you are overweight, you will burn up more calories while exercising than a person of normal weight.

5. According to studies by the Harvard School of Public Health, thirty minutes of proper exercise each day can keep off or take off as much as twenty-six pounds a year.

6. A change in diet, perhaps a change as small as taking little sugar, may be all that is necessary to bring your weight down and keep it down, especially if combined with proper exercise.

7. The most effective way to lose weight and keep it off is with a program that combines proper exercise with a sensible diet.

A *word of caution:* You should not lose more than two pounds a week unless your physician advises you to do so.

FACTS ABOUT FOOD

Food is essential to life. It is our daily source of nutrients, all those things we need for our health and well-being. Despite the fact that food is a basic need, we know very little about it. As a result, we tend to eat too much of the wrong foods. Some foods are not as nutritious as others. No one food, though, provides all the daily nutrients we need. To get all the necessary benefits, we should try to eat a balanced variety of foods.

THE MAJOR NUTRIENTS AND WHERE TO FIND THEM

Protein

After water and possibly fat, protein is the most plentiful substance in the body. The substances called enzymes, which control the processes that keep the body working, are made of protein. Protein is also part of the hemoglobin molecule in red blood cells, which carries oxygen throughout the body. The antibodies in the bloodstream that fight off disease and infection are also protein. Another important use of protein in the body is to build the muscle tissue that holds the bone structure together and provides the strength to move and work. Most Americans get more than enough protein from the meat, poultry, fish, milk, cheese, and eggs they eat. Bread and cereal are also important sources, as are soybeans, chickpeas, dry beans, and peanuts. You do not have to load up on meat, poultry, or eggs to get enough protein in your diet.

Combining cereal or vegetable foods with a little milk, cheese, or other animal protein can provide good protein in your diet. For example, eat cereal with milk, rice with fish, spaghetti and meatballs, or simply drink a glass of milk during a meal. All these combinations provide the high-quality protein the body needs.

Fats

Fats provide energy, add flavor and variety to foods, and make meals more satisfying.

Fats carry vitamins A, D, E and K and are essential parts of the structure of the cells that make up the body's tissue.

Our body fat also protects vital organs by providing a cushion around them.

Fats are plentiful in butter, margarine, shortening, salad oils, cream, most cheeses, mayonnaise, salad dressing, nuts, and bacon.

Carbohydrates

These are starches and sugars found in cereal grains, fruits, vegetables, and sugar added to foods for sweetening. Carbohydrates are the major source of energy in the diet. Wheat, oats, corn, and rice—and the foods made from them, such as bread, spaghetti, macaroni, noodles, or grits—provide starch along with other important nutrients. So, too, do potatoes, peas, dry beans, peanuts, and soybeans. Most of the other vegetables contain smaller amounts of carbohydrates.

Water

Water is a most important nutrient, standing next to air in importance. You can get along for days, even weeks, without food, but only a few days without water.

Water is necessary for digestion because nutrients are dissolved in it so they can pass through the intestinal wall and into the bloodstream for use throughout the body. Water also carries waste out of the body and helps to regulate body temperature.

The most obvious source of water is the water a person drinks, but some is produced when the body burns food for energy. Coffee and tea are mostly water, as are fruit juices and milk.

Soup is an excellent source of water, along with many fruits and vegetables. Even meat can be up to 80 percent water.

Minerals

The most abundant mineral in the body is calcium and, except for iron, it is the one most likely to be inadequate in the diet. From the age of nine, the diets of girls and women, especially, may lack as much as 25 to 30 percent of the calcium they need.

Almost all calcium, and most phosphorus, which works closely with calcium in the body, is in bones and teeth. The rest plays a vital role in tissue and body fluids. Soft tissue, or muscle, has a particularly high phosphorus content. Calcium is required for blood clotting and normal heart function. The nervous system does not work properly when calcium levels in the blood are below normal.

Most people who buy milk are stocking up on calcium supplies. In the United States we rely on milk as a basic source of calcium, and two cups of milk, or an equivalent amount of cheese or other dairy products except butter, go a long way toward supplying all the calcium needed for the day.

But milk is not the only source. Dark-green leafy vegetables, like collards, mustard greens, or turnip greens, provide some calcium; and salmon and sardines supply useful amounts of it if the very tiny bones are eaten.

Iron

Iron is another essential mineral. Women of childbearing age need more iron than men. The diets of infants and pregnant women may need special attention to see that they contain the iron needed.

Unfortunately, only a few foods provide iron in very useful amounts. But liver, heart, kidney and most lean meats are generously supplied with it. Shellfish, particularly oysters, and dark-green leafy vegetables are also sources of iron. Whole-grain and enriched breads and cereals can provide 20 to 25 percent or more of the daily iron need.

Iodine

The most important fact about iodine is that a deficiency of it can cause goiter—a swelling of the thyroid gland. The most practical ways to get enough iodine are to use iodized salt regularly and eat seafood whenever possible.

OTHER ESSENTIAL ELEMENTS

Calcium, iron and iodine are not the only minerals you need. Most of the others—zinc, copper, sodium, potassium, magnesium, and phosphorus—are widely available in so many foods that a little variety in making your choice at the grocery store easily takes care of them. Magnesium, for example, occurs in nuts, whole-grain products, dry beans, and dark-green vegetables.

Phosphorus, an element that helps protect teeth from decay—is not so readily found in food. Many metropolitan areas add minute amounts of fluorine to local sources of drinking water.

Vitamins

Scientists know of a dozen or more vitamins that you must have to enjoy good health. Ordinarily, you can get them from a well-chosen assortment of everyday foods.

A few of these vitamins are of great importance, and you should know what foods provide them.

Vitamin A

This vitamin is very important for healthy eyes and to keep skin and mucous membranes resistant to infection. Although vitamin A occurs only in foods of animal origin, the deep-yellow and dark-green vegetables and fruits supply a material called carotene, which your body can turn into vitamin A. A two-ounce serving of cooked beef liver provides more than 30,000 international units of the vitamin. That is six times more vitamin A than you would need during the day. Kidney is also an excellent source of vitamin A.

There are many other sources of vitamin A. Whole milk is a source, but skim milk doesn't have any vitamin A unless it is fortified—that is, unless vitamin A has been added to it. Cheese made from whole milk and margarine enriched with vitamin A both supply this vitamin.

The B Vitamins

Three of the best known vitamins—riboflavin, thiamin, and niacin—release the energy in food. They also have a role in the nervous system, keep the digestive system working calmly, and help maintain a healthy skin.

Vitamin B_2 (riboflavin) is easy to find and extremely important to your diet. It is plentifully supplied by meats, milk, whole-grain or enriched breads, and cereals. Organ meats (such as liver and kidney) also supply this vitamin.

A lack of thiamin (vitamin B_1) causes beriberi. Fortunately, this disease is now almost nonexistent in the United States, although it is still seen in some alcoholics. Thiamin is abundant in only a few foods. Lean pork is one. Dry beans and peas, some of the organ meats, and some nuts supply some thiamin. Whole-grain and enriched cereals and breads are also dependable sources of the vitamin.

Niacin can be found in whole-grain and enriched cereals, meat, and meat products, and in peas and beans.

Other B vitamins, such as B_6, B_{12} and folacin, are needed for normal hemoglobin, the substance in blood that carries oxygen to the tissues. B_{12} occurs in foods of animal origin. Strict vegetarians run a risk of developing the symptoms of B_{12} deficiency: soreness of the mouth and tongue, numbness and tingling in the hands and legs, anemia, and loss of coordination. Folacin is available in many foods but in small quantities.

Vitamin C

Vitamin C, ascorbic acid, is not completely understood, but it is considered to be important in maintaining the cementing material that holds body cells together.

The citrus fruit juice you have for breakfast can give you over half of the vitamin C needed for the day. In fact, the rest of the fruit and vegetables eaten during the day will provide the vitamin C required.

Potatoes and sweet potatoes provide helpful amounts of vitamin C and so do tomatoes and peppers. In addition, the green vegetables, such as broccoli, turnip greens, raw cabbage, and collards, make a contribution of vitamin C.

Vitamin D

Although few foods contain vitamin D, it is readily available in fortified milk. Sunlight makes the body produce vitamin D if it has a chance to shine directly on the skin.

Vitamin D is important in building strong bones and teeth and is needed throughout the growth period. Without it the body cannot absorb the calcium supplied by food, and for this reason milk is often fortified with vitamin D. Adults rarely need more vitamin D than they get in food and from the sun, but infants and young children sometimes do not get enough. A disease called rickets results from a lack. Children who suffer from this disease have absorbed too little calcium; their bodies cannot form strong, rigid bones. Consequently they may have enlarged joints, bowed legs, knocked knees, or beaded ribs.

On the other hand, too much vitamin D can be dangerous. This causes a calcium overload in the blood and tissues. Infants given too much vitamin D may develop calcium deposits in the kidneys and other organs and end up with permanent kidney damage.

Vitamin E

Vitamin E is known to be essential, but its exact role is not fully understood. It is abundant in vegetable oils and margarine and appears in such foods as wheat germ and lettuce. If a diet regularly includes fruits, vegetables, vegetable oil, milk, meat, and eggs, it is not lacking in vitamin E.

Vitamin K

Vitamin K is essential for blood clotting. This vitamin is found in a variety of foods such as the green and leafy vegetables, tomatoes, cauliflower, egg yolks, soybean oil, and any kind of liver.

NUTRIENTS AND ENERGY

Almost all foods provide energy, some more than others. This energy is measured in calories. Foods rich in fats, starches, or sugars contain large amounts of calories, or energy. Fat is the most concentrated source of energy. Ounce for ounce, it provides more than twice as much energy as protein or the carbohydrates. Foods that contain a lot of water, like watermelon and cucumbers, have few calories, because water, which makes up most of their weight, provides no calories and so no energy.

HOW IT ALL WORKS TOGETHER

The body can pick and choose what it needs from the nutrients in the diet and see to it that each organ or part of the body gets exactly the right amount of nutrients. But, if the diet lacks some of the needed nutrients, the body has no way to get them. The body keeps busy, working twenty-four hours a day, always building itself up, repairing itself, and discarding waste products. It needs a constant supply of nutrients to do its job, and when it receives the nutrients, it applies them where they are needed. Let us take calcium as an example. The body needs calcium to clot blood, to make the nerves and muscles function properly, and to develop bones. If your body does not receive enough calcium to do its work from the food you eat, it steals some from your bones. If the stolen calcium is not replaced, the body is in trouble, though you may not realize this fact for years. (As much as one-third of the normal amount of calcium may be withdrawn from an adult's bones before the loss shows up on an X-ray film.)

It is not only what the nutrients do once the body gets them, it is what they do with each other that makes the difference in our health and well-being. No single nutrient can function properly alone. It takes calcium to build strong bones, but that is just the beginning. Without Vitamin D, the calcium is not absorbed from the intestines. Protein is needed for the framework of the bone and to form part of every cell and all the fluids that circulate in and around the cells.

This is why nutritionists suggest eating appropriate quantities of a wide variety of foods—including milk products, meat or an alternative, fruits and vegetables, bread and cereals—in order to provide diets with all the needed nutrients. The more varied your diet, the better off you will be—tomorrow as well as today. The foods you eat must sustain you for today and help build up your body for a lifetime.

FOOD FOR ALL AGES

Regardless of age, everyone needs the same nutrients, but often in different amounts. People doing hard physical labor need more energy than those who are less active. Women need more iron than men. The six-footer needs more food than a little person, the steelworker more than the clerk. When a patient is on the mend from an illness, he may need more nutrients than when he is in good health.

One thing is certain: nutrition affects everyone from the day he is born, and actually even before he is born. Nutrients for the unborn child's growth and development come from the mother, which means that her diet during pregnancy is especially important. While parents guide their children to good eating habits, they might take a good look at their own food attitudes. If the food they do not like is never served, then the family will never get a chance to eat it, regardless of how nutritious it might be.

Changing poor food habits is usually harder than starting out with good food habits, but it can be done. The parents' example will teach children to eat foods that are not their favorites, usually without the children's ever even thinking about it. The more foods people learn to enjoy, particularly among the fruits and vegetables, the easier it will be for them to change their diets if it becomes necessary because of health problems, military service, foreign travel, or some other reason.

Before Birth

The woman who reaches childbearing age well-nourished and who maintains a good diet during pregnancy is more likely to have a healthy baby than the woman whose diet is poor.

But good nutrition during pregnancy can be a problem, particularly when expectant mothers are still teenagers. The body must cope with its own growth needs as well as the baby's. A young girl—seventeen years or younger—who is in less than the best of health when she becomes pregnant is borrowing trouble for herself and lending it to the child she carries. And it is not just the poverty-stricken teenager who faces such problems. Many a woman with enough money for a good diet copes with pregnancy in a state of semi-starvation because of the cult of slimness. Pregnancy for an older woman can also be a hazard if her body stores of nutrients are already depleted by numerous pregnancies. A woman who has always eaten well will not, ordinarily, have to make many changes in her diet because of pregnancy.

A daily diet during pregnancy should include at least two servings of lean meat, fish, poultry, or eggs; four or more servings of vegetables and fruits including some that are good sources of iron, vitamin A, and vitamin C; four servings of enriched or whole-grain breads or cereals and three or more cups of milk. Some of the milk and other foods such as margarine may be fortified with the vitamin D which is needed during pregnancy. These foods provide the extra proteins, vitamins and minerals needed to maintain the expectant mother's body and for the baby's growth. It may be hard to get all the iron and folic acid needed through food alone, and the doctor will often prescribe a supplement to supply them. Healthy women usually gain an average of twenty-four pounds during pregnancy. Pregnancy is certainly no time to lose weight; there will be time enough for that later. If a mother decides to nurse her baby, she should continue to include foods that will give her more protein, vitamins, minerals, and calories. A pint of milk and an egg added to a diet that was nutritionally adequate before pregnancy will provide all the additional protein and almost half of the vitamin A needed. Using milk as the source of extra protein also contributes to the mother's supply of fluid when nursing. The continued use of the green vegetables and fruits recommended for pregnancy will supply most of the other minerals and vitamins needed.

The Infant

A child grows and develops more rapidly during the first few years of life than at any other time. Thus good nutrition is especially important. Feeding does more than nourish the infant's body; it also helps a child to establish warm human relationships with parents.

Milk is the baby's first food, either from the mother's breast or from a bottle. Since milk supplies a large proportion of the nutrients needed during the first two years of life, the choice of kind of milk or formula must be made with care.

Human milk is custom-made for the baby, is clean as it comes from the breast, and can save a lot of work; and nursing can be a satisfying experience for both mother and baby. Human milk will ordinarily supply adequate amounts of all of the essential nutrients during the first few months of life with the exception of vitamin D, fluoride, and iron.

If commercially prepared infant formula, evaporated milk, or homogenized whole milk is used, it will probably have vitamin D added to it. If not, the baby will need to be given a vitamin D supplement. The baby needs vitamin C early in life. Human milk and commercially prepared infant formulas usually provide adequate amounts of vitamin C.

If the baby is being fed evaporated milk or cow's milk formula, then vitamin C should be given in the form of drops. Otherwise, a fresh, frozen, or canned fruit juice that is naturally rich in vitamin C or fortified with vitamin C can be used. A source of iron should also be added to the infant's diet early in infancy. Unless, the baby is receiving iron-fortified formula, the doctor may suggest using an iron-fortified infant cereal or medicinal iron, starting at one or two months of age. Whether or not a fluoride supplement is given to the infant will depend upon how much water the infant takes and the amount of fluoride in the water supply of the area.

Solid foods, such as cereals, strained fruits, and vegetables, may be added by one to three months of age. Gradually other foods such as egg yolk, strained meat, and fish are added. Be careful in choosing commercially available strained foods for baby; there are wide variations among them in the amount of calories and essential nutrients.

By the time the baby is six months old, he or she will be receiving some "table food." When seven to nine months old, a baby is usually ready for foods of coarser consistency—chopped or junior foods. By then he or she will probably be on three meals a day with mid-morning and mid-afternoon snacks.

Preschool

During the second and third years of life, the child grows much less rapidly than during the first year. Nevertheless, little children still need foods that help them grow and provide the energy they need.

The diet started in infancy should be continued with larger servings of meat, fish, and eggs, as well as fruits and vegetables, plenty of milk and whole-grain cereals and bread.

Children in this country often get less vitamin A than they need. Parents should try hard to include dark-green and yellow vegetables such as broccoli, collards, kale, carrots, sweet potatoes, and winter squash in children's meals. Butter and fortified margarine also supply generous amounts of vitamin A. Children may be short of vitamin C, because they do not eat enough citrus fruits or juice, tomatoes, raw cabbage or other foods that are rich sources of that vitamin. Fortified milk is a good source of vitamin D. The child who drinks less than one pint of milk a day may need a supplemental supply.

Preschool children may need snacks to tide them over to the next meal. Some well-chosen snacks are milk, small pieces of fruit, cut-up raw vegetables, cheese cubes, crackers spread with cottage cheese or peanut butter, and cereals. Pick snacks that carry their weight in food value; don't let sweets become the rule.

Children should be served small-sized portions and come back for "seconds" if necessary. Some children get fat because they are taught to eat more than they need, even as infants. It is possible that the habit of overeating in infancy and early childhood may continue to obesity in later years.

Between Toddler and Teen

The elementary school child needs the same kind of foods the preschooler does, but, perhaps, larger servings.

Going to school, however, calls for a routine and a schedule. Preschool children can play for a while until they feel like breakfast. Not so the school child; there are car pools, buses, and school bells to be coped with.

Going to school may be the beginning of the child's independence in choosing food. The child may need help in learning how to make wise choices. If the elementary school child is getting too plump, take a good look at the amount of exercise he is getting and at what and how much he is eating.

The Perilous Teens

There are good reasons for concern about the food habits of teenagers. Teenagers are casting off habits of childhood while still trying to find their own identities. As a result, good food habits may be lost for a while. The teenage appetite is often huge, but appetite alone is not enough to insure that the teenager will get all of the nutrients he or she needs.

During their teens, boys and girls grow at a faster rate than at any other time except infancy. A boy's nutritional requirements during the time he is becoming a man are higher than at any other time in his life. Those of a girl becoming a woman are exceeded only during pregnancy and lactation (the period following birth when the mother's breasts are manufacturing milk). So, a pregnant teenage girl has even greater nutrient needs.

A teenage boy may suddenly shoot up as much as four inches in height and gain fifteen pounds in weight in a year. A teenage girl's total gain is not usually so large, but it is considerable. Growth involves more than increases in height and weight alone. Body fat is lost while bones increase in density and muscles develop in size and strength. The endocrine glands—the glands that manufacture, or secrete, hormones, the chemical substances that control many body processes—are growing and developing.

The teen years are also a period of stress—physical and mental.

Teenage eating habits are often bad, an the reasons are not hard to find: schoo clubs, and part-time jobs keep teenage away from home at mealtime. Their eatin habits are being influenced by friends mor than by parents. Some skip breakfast be cause they don't leave enough time for i Some choose snacks that are too rich wit fats and sugars. Teenage girls sometimes e too little because they dread getting fa whether they are overweight or not.

Diets have to be planned carefully fo boys as well as girls. Both have such grea need for protein, the B vitamins, and vitami C, and, in fact, every nutrient, that they car not afford to fill up on foods that contribut empty calories alone. A teenage boy usuall winds up with a better diet than a teenag girl because his need for calories is so grea that if food is available he will eat it. Som boys, however, neglect foods containing im portant nutrients A teenage girl's need fo calories is considerably less. She is mor likely to get enough vitamin C because o her liking for salads and fruits, but her pro tein and iron intake may be low. Both boy and girls tend to neglect foods containin calcium, vitamin A, riboflavin, and iron. Du ing the growth spurt, all these nutrients ar needed for muscle, bone, and blood.

The overweight teenager may eat th same kinds of foods as his average frienc but too much of them. Rich desserts an many of the usual snack foods could be replaced with fresh fruits and vegetables. He may also be less active. Instead of a crash diet to take off pounds in a hurry, an overweight teenager should develop the well-balanced eating habits he needs for the rest of his life.

The underweight adolescent may or may not be satisfied with his state and may need help in learning how to gain weight.

It should be noted that anemia may occur in both sexes at this age, although the monthly blood loss from menstruation puts girls in the more dangerous position.

Acne, the other blight on the teen years, is usually caused by hormone changes and not by diet.

Late Teens and Early Twenties

Growth ends somewhere during the late teens and early twenties when maturity is reached and the body's slowdown begins. Compared with their youth, men and women need less protein and calcium—about two cups of milk a day provide enough calcium. Men usually get enough iron without making a special effort. Women must be sure to get extra supplies in their diets. The amount of vitamin D adults get in fortified milk is enough. Allowances for vitamins A and C are about the same as they were in younger days. Adults can get enough vitamin A in dark-green leafy vegetables or deep yellow ones eaten three times a week. The vegetables should be eaten along with the recommended daily servings of such foods as whole milk, vitamin-A-fortified skim milk, cheese made from whole milk, and butter or vitamin-A-enriched margarine. One serving of citrus fruit or juice along with other fruit and vegetables is an easy way to get enough vitamin C.

Most adults use fewer calories than they did in their teens, and weight control may be a problem. Gross overweight usually leads to medical problems, so, generally, an adult should try to maintain for the rest of his life the weight considered normal for him at age twenty-five. This means that the right amount of food at thirty may be too much at forty. Calorie counting becomes necessary. A mere twenty extra calories a day could add two pounds of weight in a year. What's two pounds? It is exactly eighty extra pounds between the ages of twenty-five and sixty-five.

Adults must make some choices about which foods to limit. Such foods as pastries, cakes, salad dressings, gravies, and nuts, if eaten frequently, may supply too many calories for many people. Frying adds fat, no matter how well the food is drained.

Sugar, candies, syrup, jellies, soft drinks, and alcohol add calories but few nutrients to the diet. Of course, cakes, dressings, jams and candy make the diet more interesting but, when they are used, be sure to compensate for the extra calories by reducing the food portions. Foods such as meats, milk, fruits, vegetables, and cereals or bread are necessary; the need for vitamins, minerals, and protein continues even though calories are being reduced.

Be careful when you are counting calories. A diet that furnishes 1,500 calories a day could be lacking in some important nutrient, depending on the choices made. The easiest way to bring the total nutrient value of a low-calorie diet up to standard is to be sure that each food does double duty. For a mid-morning pickup, fresh fruit or juice can provide vitamins C and A that would be lacking in pastry, and, by the same token, a plate of fresh fruit, instead of apple pie for dessert, can provide vitamins C and A with relatively fewer calories.

Eating in Later Years

The process of aging begins the moment a person is conceived. It is hard to say exactly when youth becomes middle age, or middle age becomes old age. Calendars tell only part of the story.

Some men and women in their eighties are still going strong; some are feeble in their sixties. The cells of an older person's body undergo changes, and some of the cells are damaged. The body's organs don't function as well. Vision is not as clear, hearing is not as sharp, and the digestive systems may act up.

The older person's condition is affected b[y] all the accidents, infection, and other ha[z]ards of living that he has experienced durin[g] his lifetime. This is when the results of poor diet through the years can be seen. A[ll] the nutrients that have been supplied, or n[ot] supplied, are giving the cells more, or les[s] strength to fight the aging process and di[s]ease. The food likes and dislikes develope[d] over the years can become barriers to goo[d] nutrition. Older people also need fewer ca[l]ories. Men and women fifty-five to seventy[-]five years old need 150 to 200 fewer calorie[s] per day than when they were thirty-five t[o] fifty-five, but their needs for essential n[u]trients are unchanged. It is more importan[t] than ever for each food to do double dut[y.] There is not much room for low-nutrien[t,] high-calorie food.

Old age, like the teen years, is a time [of] learning to live with changes. Often th[e] changes are serious and tiring. The strains [of] old age may be made worse by changes i[n] living patterns. The eating habits of the e[l]derly can be influenced by loss of teeth, re[]tirement, reduced income, moving out of [a] familiar house or neighborhood, or the num[]ber of people with whom they live.

NUTRITIONAL LABELING

It is one thing to know what nutrients w[e] need; it is another to get them. Of the eigh[t] thousand or more items in a large food stor[e] today, half or more are packaged foods. In[]

dustry and government, therefore, have cooperated in providing a nutrient listing on packaged foods.

This new development, "nutritional labeling," represents a major change in food labeling. Foods with nutritional labeling have a *Nutritional Information* panel on their packages, which gives the consumer the serving size, number of servings in the container, and the calories, protein, carbohydrate, and fat per serving. In addition, the statement gives the percentage of the U.S. Recommended Daily Allowance (U.S. RDA) of protein and seven major vitamins and minerals per serving. Additional nutrients may also be listed, along with information on sodium, cholesterol, and unsaturated fat.

Nutritional labeling is voluntary except when a nutrient is added or a special nutritional or dietetic claim is made, and then the label must provide nutritional labeling. The standard for declaring the nutrients, the U.S. Recommended Daily Allowance (U.S. RDA), has been developed by the Food and Drug Administration of the Department of Health, Education and Welfare from the Recommended Daily Dietary Allowance set by the National Academy of Sciences' Food and Nutrition Board. The National Academy has developed twenty-four sets of allowances covering different age groups.

Nutritional labeling provides a means of identifying the specific nutrients and the nutrient content of foods. It also provides nutrient information for those new fabricated products that often do not seem to fit into traditional food guides.

People interested in weight control or those on special diets for other reasons will find the information helpful in selecting the proper foods. Nutritional labeling, in conjunction with the traditional methods of selecting a diet of many kinds of foods or a diet based on the basic four food groups, can help the consumer improve and maintain the quality of his diet.

A DAILY FOOD GUIDE

There are four basic food groups:

Meats
Vegetables and fruits
Milk
Bread and cereals

Meat Group

Foods Included: Beef; veal; lamb; pork; variety meats, such as liver, heart, kidney. Poultry and eggs. Fish and shellfish.

As alternatives—dry beans, dry peas, lentils, nuts, peanuts, peanut butter.

Amounts Recommended: Choose two or more servings every day. Count as a serving: two to three ounces of lean cooked meat, poultry, or fish—all without bone.

One egg, one-half cup cooked dry beans, dry peas, or lentils, or two tablespoons peanut butter may replace one-half serving of meat.

Vegetable-Fruit Group

Foods Included: All vegetables and fruits. This guide emphasizes those that are valuable sources of vitamin C and vitamin A.

Sources of vitamin C:

Good sources—grapefruit or grapefruit juice; orange or orange juice; cantaloupe; guava; mango; papaya; fresh strawberries; broccoli; brussels sprouts; green pepper; sweet red pepper.

Fair sources—honeydew melon; lemon; tangerine or tangerine juice; watermelon; asparagus tips; raw cabbage; collards; garden cress; kale; kohlrabi; mustard greens; potatoes and sweet potatoes cooked in the jacket; spinach; tomatoes or tomato juice; turnip greens.

Sources of vitamin A:

Dark-green and deep yellow vegetables and a few fruits: apricots, broccoli, cantaloupe, carrots, chard, collards, cress, kale, mango, persimmon, pumpkin, spinach, sweet potatoes, turnip greens and other dark-green leafy vegetables, winter squash.

Amounts Recommended: Choose four or more servings every day, including:

One serving of a good source of vitamin C or two servings of a fair source.

One serving, at least every other day, of a good source of vitamin A. If the food chosen for vitamin C is also a good source of vitamin A, the additional serving of a vitamin A food may be omitted.

Count as one serving: one-half cup of vegetable or fruit; or a portion as ordinarily served, such as one medium orange or potato, half a medium grapefruit or cantaloupe or the juice of one lemon.

Milk Group

Foods Included: Milk—fluid whole; evaporated; skim; dry; buttermilk. Cheese—cottage; cream; Cheddar-type, natural or processed; ice cream; yogurt.

Amounts Recommended: Some milk every day for everyone.

Recommended amounts are given below in terms of eight-ounce cups of whole fluid milk:

Children under 9 .... 2 to 3
Children 9 to 12 .... 3 or more
Teenagers .... 4 or more
Adults .... 2 or more
Pregnant mothers .... 4 or more
Nursing mothers .... 4 or more

Part or all of the milk may be fluid skim milk, buttermilk, evaporated milk, or dry milk.

Other milk products, such as cheese, ice cream or yogurt, may replace part of the milk. The amount it will take to replace a given amount of milk is figured on the basis of calcium content. Common portions of cheese, yogurt, and ice cream and their milk equivalents in calcium are:

1-inch cube Cheddar-type cheese	= ½ cup milk
½ cup yogurt	= ½ cup milk
½ cup cottage cheese	= ⅓ cup milk
2 tablespoons cream cheese	= 1 tablespoon milk

Bread-Cereal Group

Foods Included: All breads and cereals that are whole-grain, enriched, or restored; check labels to be sure.

Specifically, this group includes: breads; cooked cereals; ready-to-eat cereals; corn-meal; crackers; flour; grits; macaroni and spaghetti; noodles; rice; rolled oats; and quick breads and other baked goods if made with whole-grain or enriched flour.

Bulgur and parboiled rice and wheat can also be included in this group.

Amounts Recommended: Choose four or more servings daily. If cereals are not eaten, have an extra serving of breads or baked goods, which will make at least five servings from this group daily.

Count as one serving: 1 slice of bread; 1 ounce ready-to-eat cereal; one-half to three-quarter cup cooked cereal, cornmeal, grits, macaroni, noodles, rice, or spaghetti.

Other Foods

To round out meals and meet energy needs, almost everyone will use some foods not specified in the four food groups. Such foods include: unenriched, refined breads, cereals, and flours; sugars; butter; margarine; other fats. These often are ingredients in a recipe or are added to other foods during preparation or at the dinner table. *Try to include some vegetable oil among the fats used.*

Some foods also fall into several groups—pizza, for example. It is desirable, however, to have the proper number of servings from each of the groups in the course of the day.

The same food guide can work for everyone. The difference is only in the quantity—more of everything for the ravenous teenager, and choices with fewer calories for the dieting adult; more of certain foods for the pregnant woman, and less of these foods for her husband.

Don't neglect breakfast. Many people skip breakfast, but scientists have found much evidence that a good breakfast can make a person more alert and productive throughout the morning. A good breakfast can provide a good start to meeting the daily nutrient needs.

THE VALUE OF PROCESSED FOODS

Fresh or frozen? Canned or dried? Instant or from scratch? Which foods have the nutrients? Which do not? They all do. All foods have their place. And virtually all food in its place is good food. Some foods are safer to use when they are processed. Some are more appealing when fresh. Packaged, pasteurized, fortified milk has been around so long no one thinks of it anymore as processed food, but it is. Because it is pasteurized, milk is now safe to drink. Unpasteurized milk may carry disease-producing germs.

Whole-grain bread and cereals retain the germ and outer layers of grain where the B vitamins concentrate. Milling wheat to white flour refines them out. Since many people seem to prefer white bread, it is wise to choose the enriched product because of added nutrients.

Brown rice has food value that unenriched, polished white rice does not; enriched, parboiled, or converted rice retains most, though not all, of the nutrients.

Buy the mix or do it yourself? It is all the same nutritionally if the ingredients listed on the label are used in the same amounts and are the same as the ingredients you would use doing it yourself.

Foods in the frozen-food case offer as much food value as those in the produce section of the store. It just depends on which foods one prefers and the cost factor. Any loss of vitamin C in frozen fruits is negligible. The blanching process does, however, reduce slightly the vitamin C and some of the other water-soluble vitamins and minerals in frozen vegetables.

Properly packaged frozen meat, poultry and fish carry the same food value as do fresh. Fresh or raw foods are not necessarily better than canned or frozen ones. It depends on how they are handled. The vitamin C value of frozen, reconstituted orange juice is the same as the juice squeezed fresh from oranges. Leafy, dark-green vegetables and broccoli packed in crushed ice keep practically all of their vitamin C on their way to market. Left in the refrigerator for five days or so, they lose about half of it. Cooking will also cause losses. Although the loss may be great, these vegetables contain large amounts of vitamins, and they still provide generous amounts of vitamin C and vitamin A when they are eaten. Raw cabbage, on the other hand, stores well. It holds its vitamin C well even at room temperature. Sweet potatoes actually improve in storage. The vitamin A value of sweet potatoes increases during the maturing period before they reach the retail store. Berries need tender care. They lose their vitamin C in a hurry if they are cut or bruised.

Water-soluble vitamins do just what their name implies: they dissolve in water; and if excess water is used in cooking and then discarded, a loss occurs. Leftovers and foods cooked ahead of time may save time, but they can have a loss in food value. Cooked vegetables lose about one-fourth of their vitamin C after about a day in the refrigerator. They lose about one-third after two days. Careful planning is needed if food values are to be protected.

When meat or poultry is stewed, some of the B vitamins end up in the stock—that is, the left-over liquid. With a kettle of stock you have a flavorful liquid in which to cook rice, or to use as the liquid base for scalloped or creamed dishes, or to make a nourishing soup.

Cold makes the difference for frozen foods. Most frozen foods should be stored far below the 32°F point to retain the vitamin C.

Acid foods like orange and tomato juice, however, hold on to their vitamin C tenaciously.

Frozen concentrated orange juice that is kept at 32°F loses only 5 percent of its vitamin C in a year.

This is not true for most other foods. At 0°F, frozen beans, broccoli, cauliflower, and spinach lose one-third to three-fourths of their vitamin C in a year. If you cannot get your freezer to 0°F or below, remember that some stored foods will not hold their best nutritive value. It is wise to buy them in smaller quantities and not hold them as long.

THE MANY WAYS OF EATING

Americans pick and choose their diets from the traditions of the whole world. Whether it is pumpkin pie or Chinese fried rice, much of our food has a special history and we are the richer for it. Our food has all sorts of social, geographical, and cultural traditions— baseball and hot dogs, San Francisco and Chinese food, New Orleans and shrimp gumbo, the Southwest and chili. All have become American traditions.

Everyone needs the same nutrients, but we can take them as we like them. Protein is important to us all. If, for example, our heritage is Mexican-American, we can get a healthy amount of protein at a low cost in such dishes as refried beans.

Or consider iron. Jewish mothers, like all women, have a special need for iron in their diets. Of the many Jewish foods, one of the most popular is a good source of iron—chopped chicken livers.

Families from Puerto Rico need milk, as everyone else does. They get a fair amount of it in *café con leche* or in *flan*. Hankering for soul food, you may find yourself fixing grits and turnip greens, and when you do you are serving up a large portion of iron, vitamin A, B vitamins, and vitamin C.

Every cultural tradition allows for enough good food for people to be healthy as well as happy at the dinner table.

Traditional eating patterns and habits may suffer a change on their way to this country, or from farm to city, but the nourishment in the food itself remains the same. Rice, for example, is a mainstay at Puerto Rican tables; it is just as important when the family moves to New York. But there are times when tradition itself changes, catching the homemaker unaware. Older Mexican-Americans like their tortillas made from cornmeal. Their children often prefer them made from wheat flour, and thus they lose out on the calcium that attached itself to the corn in the processing.

For all its people, however, the United States has one of the best food supplies in the world, whether measured in terms of quantity, quality, variety, or availability.

If your diet contains a good variety of foods, whether fresh or packaged, meats and vegetables, milk, cereals, and grains, fruits and cheeses in the necessary amounts, good nutrition will take care of itself.

FOOD AND NUTRITION BOARD,

NATIONAL ACADEMY OF SCIENCES—

NATIONAL RESEARCH COUNCIL RECOMMENDED

DAILY DIETARY ALLOWANCES,[a] Revised 1974

Designed for the maintenance of good nutrition

of practically all healthy people in the U.S.A.

	Age (Years)	Weight (kg)	Weight (lbs)	Height (cm)	Height (in)	Energy (kcal)[b]	Protein (g)	FAT-SOLUBLE VITAMINS		
								Vitamin A Activity (RE)[c]	Vitamin A Activity (IU)	Vitamin D (IU)
Infants	0.0–0.5	6	14	60	24	kg × 117	kg × 2.2	420[d]	1,400	400
	0.5–1.0	9	20	71	28	kg × 108	kg × 2.0	400	2,000	400
Children	1–3	13	28	86	34	1,300	23	400	2,000	400
	4–6	20	44	110	44	1,800	30	500	2,500	400
	7–10	30	66	135	54	2,400	36	700	3,300	400
Males	11–14	44	97	158	63	2,800	44	1,000	5,000	400
	15–18	61	134	172	69	3,000	54	1,000	5,000	400
	19–22	67	147	172	69	3,000	54	1,000	5,000	400
	23–50	70	154	172	69	2,700	56	1,000	5,000	—
	51+	70	154	172	69	2,400	56	1,000	5,000	—
Females	11–14	44	97	155	62	2,400	44	800	4,000	400
	15–18	54	119	162	65	2,100	48	800	4,000	400
	19–22	58	128	162	65	2,100	46	800	4,000	400
	23–50	58	128	162	65	2,000	46	800	4,000	—
	51+	58	128	162	65	1,800	46	800	4,000	—
Pregnant						+300	+30	1,000	5,000	400
Lactating						+500	+20	1,200	6,000	400

a The allowances are intended to provide for individual variations among most normal persons as they live in the United States under usual environmental stresses. Diets should be based on a variety of common foods in order to provide other nutrients for which human requirements have been less well defined.

b Kilojoules (KJ) = 4.2 × kcal.

c Retinol equivalents.

d Assumed to be all as retinol in milk during the first six months of life. All subsequent intakes are assumed to be half as retinol and half as β-carotene when calculated from international units. As retinol equivalents, three-fourths are as retinol and one-fourth as β-carotene.

	WATER-SOLUBLE VITAMINS						MINERALS					
Ascorbic Acid (mg)	Folacin^f (μg)	Niacin^g (mg)	Riboflavin (mg)	Thiamin (mg)	Vitamin B_6 (mg)	Vitamin B_{12} (μg)	Calcium (mg)	Phosphorus (mg)	Iodine (μg)	Iron (mg)	Magnesium (mg)	Zinc (mg)
35	50	5	0.4	0.3	0.3	0.3	360	240	35	10	60	3
35	50	8	0.6	0.5	0.4	0.3	540	400	45	15	70	5
40	100	9	0.8	0.7	0.6	1.0	800	800	60	15	150	10
40	200	12	1.1	0.9	0.9	1.5	800	800	80	10	200	10
40	300	16	1.2	1.2	1.2	2.0	800	800	110	10	250	10
45	400	18	1.5	1.4	1.6	3.0	1,200	1,200	130	18	350	15
45	400	20	1.8	1.5	2.0	3.0	1,200	1,200	150	18	400	15
45	400	20	1.8	1.5	2.0	3.0	800	800	140	10	350	15
45	400	18	1.6	1.4	2.0	3.0	800	800	130	10	350	15
45	400	16	1.5	1.2	2.0	3.0	800	800	110	10	350	15
45	400	16	1.3	1.2	1.6	3.0	1,200	1,200	115	18	300	15
45	400	14	1.4	1.1	2.0	3.0	1,200	1,200	115	18	300	15
45	400	14	1.4	1.1	2.0	3.0	800	800	100	18	300	15
45	400	13	1.2	1.0	2.0	3.0	800	800	100	18	300	15
45	400	12	1.1	1.0	2.0	3.0	800	800	80	10	300	15
60	800	+2	+0.3	+0.3	2.5	4.0	1,200	1,200	125	18+^h	450	20
80	600	+4	+0.5	+0.3	2.5	4.0	1,200	1,200	150	18	450	25

e Total vitamin E activity, estimated to be 80 percent as α-tocopherol and 20 percent other tocopherols.

f The folacin allowances refer to dietary sources as determined by *Lactobacillus casei* assay. Pure forms of folacin may be effective in doses less than one-fourth of the recommended dietary allowance.

g Although allowances are expressed as niacin, it is recognized that on the average 1 mg of niacin is derived from each 60 mg of dietary tryptophan.

h This increased requirement cannot be met by ordinary diets; therefore, the use of supplemental iron is recommended.

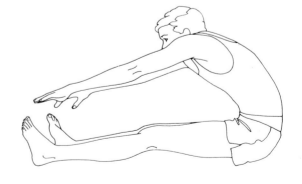